I had just had surgery that morning for colon cancer and was still adjusting to my new diagnosis when you gave me a session of gentle touch that evening in the hospital. The experience was very spiritual and healing. While you were with me, I felt great presence and thanksgiving.

As you touched each part of my body, my thoughts formed a mantra. Each segment represents one of the areas of my body you touched:

> May I be embraced by the presence of the holy;
>
> May I be centered in thought, word, and deed;
>
> May I be open to this day of joy and thanksgiving;
>
> May I give the gift of love to others in all that I do and
>   may I be open to receive love from others;
>
> May I walk in my own path;
>
> May I be physically, mentally, and spiritually strong so that
>   I may truly be present to the world around me;
>
> May I be open to the Spirit of Life whose roots uphold me
>   and whose wings set me free.
>
> — Dr. Melissa L. Buchan

DEDICATED TO MARCELLA MACDONALD, MOTHER, TEACHER, GUIDE, SOUNDING BOARD, AND THE ONE I CAN TELL MY STORIES TO.

ACKNOWLEDGMENTS

In addition to my mother, many others were instrumental in bringing this project to fruition:

Mary Bothwell, whose encouragement and writing lessons were essential; Harriet Anani, Clinical Nurse Specialist in oncology, who guided and mentored me as we established OHSU's massage program, answered innumerable questions even after leaving the job, and proofed parts of the manuscript; Ivy Nelson, OHSU Volunteer Coordinator—her idea started it all; Elizabeth Bothwell, whose computer wizardry brought my vision to life on the page; and Thierry and Karin Bogliolo of Findhorn Press for their devotion to making the world a better place through books.

Many Registered Nurses filled the gaps in my knowledge: Kay Slick, Sandi Kelleher, Tom Pryor, Lori Andreas, Debbie Johnson, Susan Lien, Patti Pahlka, Evelyn Brady, and Diane Charmley. Thanks to Physical Therapist Karen Garnett, OHSU pharmacist Joe Bubalo for researching chemotherapies, pediatric oncologist Greg Thomas, M.D. and Carol Brownlow for input on the metastasis chapter. Credit must go to Karen Gibson for inadvertently giving me the title to chapter four, "Piecing the Body Together," during a phone conversation. Reiki Masters Sheila King and Phil Morgan, along with hospice nurse Alina Egerman, Anne Jackson of the Oregon Hospice Association, and Kik Lovegren, massage therapist for Washington County Hospice, spent hours talking to me about being with people who are dying.

Thanks to the massage therapists and students who were willing to be photographed as they worked: Devon Mathews, Joan Pinkert, and Elizabeth Thorpe from Oregon School of Massage; Sara Barney, Trudy Kmetova, Lynn Parrish, Tina Schafer, and Katy VonAtta from Cedar Mountain Center for Massage in Vancouver, WA; and Jane Galen from Hopewell House in Portland, OR.

Thanks also to photographer Don Hamilton whose enthusiasm, generosity, and friendship made the photo shoots easy and comfortable.

And finally, I acknowledge the students in the hospital massage classes. We have learned and grown together.

13428

moore

M[ ]DS

MASSAG[ ] CANCER

Cumbria   **CUMBRIA LIBRARY SERVICES**

COUNTY COUNCIL

This book is due to be returned on or before the last date above. It may be renewed by personal application, post or telephone, if not in demand.

C.L.18

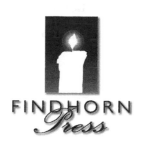

FINDHORN
Press

IMPORTANT, PLEASE READ:

Prior to initiating the use of massage or any other touch modalities, consult with the patient's doctor. *Medicine Hands* is designed to be a resource, it is not a substitute for medical advice. Different state or municipal licensing boards have jurisdiction over the practice of massage. These regulating bodies may have a policy or recommendation with regard to massaging people with cancer. Practitioners should become knowledgeable about these regulations by contacting the licensing board.

Publisher's Cataloging-in-Publication
(Provided by Quality Books, Inc.)

MacDonald, Gayle, 1950-
   Medicine Hands : massage therapy for people with cancer / Gayle MacDonald
   p. cm.
   Includes biographical references and index.
   ISBN 1-899171-77-0

   1. Cancer--Palliative treatment.   2. Massage therapy.
I. Title.

   RC271.P38M33 1999   916.99'40622
                 QBI99-509

British Library Cataloguing-in-Publication Data

A catalogue record for this book
is available from
the British Library.

Photography by Don Hamilton
Cover design by Phoenix Graphics, Winter Haven, Florida.

Printed and bound by Patterson Printing, USA.

Published by

Findhorn Press

The Park, Findhorn,
Forres IV36 3TY
Scotland
Tel 01309 690582 - 0800 389 9395
Fax 01309 690036

P.O. Box 13939
Tallahassee
Florida 32317-3939, USA
Tel 850 893 2920 - 877 390 4425
Fax 850 893 3442

e-mail: info@findhornpress.com
findhornpress.com

Table of Contents

Preface

One afternoon I received a long-distance telephone call from a terrified massage therapist. The practitioner had massaged a client that day who failed to indicate on the intake form that she had a history of cancer. Only after the session did the woman mention it. Even though the recipient had been declared cancer free years before, the therapist panicked. She was deeply frightened that she might have done something to cause harm. Like many massage practitioners, she had been taught as a student that cancer is **always** a contraindication for massage.

Medicine Hands grew out of my desire to soothe the fears and provide encouragement for those like the panicked therapist who are frightened to work with clients who have cancer. While it is true that a typical session of Swedish Massage, Shiatsu, or Trigger Point Therapy may be inappropriate for some patients, by adapting techniques or using another gentler, non-invasive modality, the benefits of touch can be experienced by all oncology patients. The goal of this book is to instill the idea that touch can **always** be safely administered to cancer patients, regardless of the severity of their condition. Hopefully it will provide the knowledge, encouragement, reassurance, and guidance to help practitioners focus on how they can enhance the lives of those living with cancer instead of concentrating on monsters in the closet.

This book is the result of working with cancer patients and supervising massage students for four years on the oncology unit at Oregon Health Sciences University (OHSU). OHSU is a large teaching and research hospital, which means many of the patients are referred there because of severe or unusual forms of cancer. The students and I therefore have been blessed to assist a number of very sick people and to witness the undeniable benefits of massage in a wide variety of situations, for patients just out of surgery, those with bone marrow transplants, people admitted for bowel problems due to the side effects of pain medication, or patients who have lost part of a colon, a kidney, breast, lung, arm, or part of their faces. We have found ways to touch those healing from radiation burns, struggling for breath, or enduring a bone marrow biopsy.

Skilled touch is beneficial at nearly every stage of the cancer experience, during hospitalization, the pre- or postoperative period, in the out-patient clinic, during chemotherapy and radiation, recovery at home, remission or cure, and in the end stages of life. Not only are physical needs addressed, but emotional, social, and spiritual ones as well. Receiving comforting, attentive bodywork reminds the patient that the body can still be a source of pleasure. As they relax, pain, fatigue, and nausea diminish. Touch reminds them they are still lovable and worthwhile. For a moment, this person, who may be disfigured, lonely, or without hope, feels whole again.

A vast amount of information already exists relative to working with the ill and dying, such as breathing and relaxation techniques, exploring and coping with grief, communication skills, the use of intuition, or compassionate touch techniques. However, *Medicine Hands* is a presentation of information not readily found in other texts. It does not attempt to replicate or improve upon what is available from other sources, but confines itself mainly to that which adds to the knowledge base with respect to cancer patients.

This book is for both professional and non-professional bodyworkers wishing to work with clients, friends, or family members. No attempt is made to teach any style of bodywork or touch techniques. It is assumed that the reader is already skilled in a chosen modality, whether it is Reiki, Swedish Massage, Shiatsu, Polarity Therapy, Therapeutic Touch, Reflexology, or any of the multitude of techniques.

Medicine Hands is for the private practitioner who wants to know how to approach a client with IV sites or to understand how steroids relate to bodywork. It is for the massage therapist seeking data to substantiate the benefits of massage for proposals to hospital boards. It is for the lay practitioner whose friend has lost hair, energy, and appetite from chemotherapy. It is for the massage therapist who has been trained to believe that all massage will contribute to metastasis. It is for the social worker or pastoral counselor who never before considered massage as an intervention for loneliness or for the burnout of a caregiver. And it is a resource for the nurse and physician in determining what kind of touch is possible and appropriate for their patients.

The book's title came from the comment of a nursing assistant to whom I was giving a seated massage. "You have medicine hands," she said. In Native American cosmology, medicine exists in everything – the wind, animals, the sea, or even a rock. Something is medicinal if it creates a connection with the energy of the universe. Personal power comes from connecting with energies that bring to us that which is needed for healing. These medicinal energies are unique to each individual. They may be in the breath, the flute, the bear, or the hands.

We all have medicine to offer through our hands. Touch is a way of connecting with the healing energies of the universe, of creating a conduit that helps patients re-connect with themselves. A bodyworker friend has the following quote on her office wall:

No single therapeutic agent can be compared in efficiency with this familiar but perfect tool… The Human Hand. If half as much research had been expended on the principles governing manual treatment as upon pharmacology, the hand would be esteemed today on a par with drugs in acceptability and power.

—J. Madison Taylor, M.D., 1908

Gayle MacDonald can be reached via email on <medhands@hotmail.com>.

Chapter 1
Introduction

The most recent statistics from the American Cancer Society regarding invasive cancers are extremely sobering. At some point, usually in later life, over one in three American women will be affected, and nearly one out of two men.[1] As they travel the road of their cancer experience, patients will have pain that the best medications cannot totally alleviate, their self-image will be shattered, they will suffer from lost relationships, anxiety about the future, or have a sore back from lying too long on a guerney. The simple act of attentive touch, whether it be slow, easy effleurage, Reiki, gentle Shiatsu, or CranioSacral Therapy, is good medicine for the multitude of physical and emotional discomforts that accompany cancer and its treatment. Touch therapists have the opportunity to enhance the health and quality of life for clients, family, and friends who are affected by this disease. In their hands is the potential to ease pain, nausea, or fatigue, to rebuild hope, to provide a forum for expressing feelings, or to give a moment of relaxation.

Cancer is the most feared of all diseases, which carries with it a sense of impending death, stigma, and isolation.

NOLA MARTEN, R.N.
AND BETTY DAVIES, R.N.

Although some bodyworkers are comfortable with and knowledgeable about massaging people with cancer or a history of it, many in the massage community are in a state of confusion and fear. Often times, therapists who have been instilled with apprehension during their formal training, turn these patients away. Some practitioners leave school with a phobia about even touching oncology patients. One massage therapist recounted a story about her mother who had been diagnosed with liver cancer. Mother asked the daughter to rub her feet, but the daughter had been so thoroughly indoctrinated in school to never massage a cancer patient that she told her mother she couldn't touch her because of the cancer.

An attitude of trepidation is injurious to patients and practitioners. It is harmful to patients because it denies them access to a service which is beneficial and further stigmatizes an already branded group. Practitioners are damaged because of an atmosphere of apprehension, so even when bodyworkers do embark on working with cancer patients, they often do so with a lack of confidence that carries through their being and into their hands. One therapist tells how she hesitantly agreed to massage a young man dying from cancer. As she worked, her feelings fluctuated between a fear of what she was doing and excitement at the way in which the patient was benefiting from the touch.

EXAMINING THE FEAR

Where does this attitude originate? The specialists who care for oncology patients are not the present-day source, as most are supportive of touch for their patients. Granted, cancer experts caution against deep bodywork and massaging the site of tumors, but it is mostly within the bodywork community that this broad-based fear is perpetuated. Beliefs about cancer and massage seem to be predominantly influenced by the various governmental bodies that regulate massage, professional bodywork organizations, and training institutions, rather than by experts in the field of oncology.

The warning about cancer and massage has been passed down without examination from one generation of bodyworker to the next. But it is incongruent with actual practice and knowledge. More and more hospitals are initiating massage programs that include or even focus on cancer patients. For example, a few hospitals that provide massage for oncology patients are the Southwest Washington Medical Center (Vancouver, WA), the Baptist Regional Cancer Center (Knoxville, TN), Boulder Community Hospital (Boulder, CO), the Geffen Cancer Center and Research Institute (Vero Beach, FL), and the Cancer Treatment Center (Tulsa, OK). Even the American Cancer Society and the National Cancer Institute advocate massage and pressure as ways to relieve pain without medicine in a pamphlet titled "Questions and Answers about Pain Control." In addition, the patient guide "Managing Cancer Pain," provided by the U.S. Department of Health and Human Services, also lists massage, pressure, vibration, and hot or cold packs as adjuvant pain therapies.

Perhaps the belief that bodywork is contraindicated for cancer patients came about during a time when Swedish Massage was the primary modality being practiced and the term "massage" was equated with deep, brisk, forceful work. The number of bodywork modalities, especially gentle, non-invasive ones, is now so vast that to define "massage" in such narrow terms exacerbates the problem. By expanding the notion of "massage" to mean any systematic form of touch which gives comfort or promotes good health[2], bodyworkers

BASIC CANCER VOCABULARY

Adjuvant Therapy The use of another form of treatment in addition to the primary one.

Benign A non-invasive tumor.

Cancerous A tumor that has the capacity to be invasive.

Invasive The ability of a tumor to spread into healthy tissue either locally or at a distance.

Malignant An invasive tumor.

Metastases The secondary growths that originated in another part of the body.

Metastatic Cancer that has spread from the original site to a secondary one.

Neoplasm Another term for tumor. It literally means new growth.

Oncology The study of tumors.

Tumor A new and abnormal growth of tissue.

Source: Thomas, C.L., ed. *Taber's Cyclopedic Medical Dictionary.* Philadelphia: F.A. Davis Co., 1993.

can explore new possibilities when working with cancer patients rather than dwell upon groundless fears.

The major apprehension of many bodyworkers is that massage, or even touch, will cause cancer cells to be released from the primary tumor and metastasize to a distant site. Students usually leave school with a simplistic view of this highly complex process and with notions that are based on emotion rather than knowledge. Bodywork practitioners have reported a fear that they will kill a cancer patient by massaging them, will cause the tumor cells to go wild, or at the very least will injure them. The goal of *Medicine Hands* is to instill the idea that a safe way can always be found to provide touch to cancer patients despite their condition. Oncology patients need never be denied compassionate, nurturing touch. By adapting techniques, modifying pressure, or switching modalities, patients can receive bodywork appropriate to their medical condition.

This does not mean bodyworkers should throw caution to the wind and work without restraint, nor should the seriousness of metastatic disease be minimized. Without a doubt it is an ominous threat. Metastatic tumors, rather than the primary ones, are most often the cause of death. [3] The reason for this is that in most cases neoplasms develop slowly and silently over the course of decades. By the time patients present to their physicians with a palpable tumor, the metastatic process has already begun. It is estimated that 30 percent of patients with solid tumors already have metastases by the time of the initial diagnosis. Another 20 to 30 percent have micrometastases at the time of initial treatment.[4] The cellular processes involved in metastatic disease occur while patients go about the most sedate of activities, such as reading, sleeping, or cooking. Refusing all massage to people with cancer will not stop the disease from spreading, but it will deny them the many benefits bodywork has to offer during this stressful time.

While it would be ludicrous to suggest that massage is a cure for cancer, the research has shown a variety of touch modalities to positively affect symptoms related to cancer or side effects from treatment, such as nausea, fatigue, insomnia, edema, and pain. Studies of hospitalized patients who received Swedish Massage have also shown it to improve mood, induce relaxation, and decrease anxiety and the sense of isolation. People living with cancer reported that weekly massage improved their quality of life. They had more energy, were better able to perform daily activities, and had less psychological distress. Lymphatic drainage therapies have proven useful in reducing the lymphedema that sometimes occurs after a mastectomy and Myofascial Release has successfully been used to relieve the pain of fibrosis after a lumpectomy and radiation.

For many touch therapists, working with cancer patients is an essential part of their own healing and journey toward wholeness. Because bodywork is one component of a holistic health model, it is imperative that its practitioners take the same approach. Bodyworkers are encouraged to make their experience as practitioners holistic,

Possibly more than any other medical specialty, oncology needs the soothing, caring attention of complementary practices. It is a merger that can greatly enhance patients' quality of life, as well as their satisfaction with cancer medicine.

— BARRIE CASSILETH, PH.D.
AND CHRISTOPHER CHAPMAN, B.A.

protocols yet exist regarding the administration of massage to people with cancer. Other bodyworkers who practice in this arena may follow slightly different guidelines than those presented in this book. Hopefully, *Medicine Hands* will start a discussion that eventually leads to a more standard approach.

PERSONAL NOTE

When I began giving massage to people with cancer, it was in the hospital, and I knew next to nothing. I was not trained as a nurse, physical therapist, or social worker. I was a teacher and a bodyworker who had no formal preparation for hospital work, but had a desire to be with the seriously ill and a fearlessness about asking questions. I learned from scratch, making more than a few mistakes in the process, which greatly helped when it was time to assist massage students in learning to apply their bodywork skills in the hospital setting. My lack of formal training in health care was beneficial in teaching massage students and in writing this book. This allowed me to experience the hospital and the patients much as the students would and to know exactly what the average bodyworker needed instruction in.

I wasn't completely without advantages when embarking on this path. My mother is a nurse, and I was conceived at about the time she started her first nursing job, which was in a hospital. During those nine months I was being acclimatized unconsciously, in utero, to the hospital milieu. Strange as it may sound, being around sick people seemed natural.

For all of my professional life my mother has filled the gaps in my education. She has been a mentor and teacher whom I could call upon day and night to answer the little questions that arise in the course of a day's work. This has been a huge blessing. Even after twenty-five years of various health-related teaching assignments, I still phone my mother at least once a week with a question. Not everyone is so lucky. In case your mother isn't a nurse, and you have no one to help fill the gaps in your education, I have tried to write this book in sufficient detail to answer your "nuts and bolts" questions.

Often times before bodyworkers start their training, they massage family, friends, and lovers with a joyful innocence. Massage school can take that away, replacing it with fears about causing harm, lawsuits, or how to correctly relate to clients. Being mindful of these issues is important, but a balance must be struck so that the pure delight of giving touch to another human being does not get lost. It is easy when presenting material about disease to create fear instead of confidence. I have tried to present this information in a way that will give you the assurance to proceed ahead, mixed with an appropriate amount of caution.

It has been an honor and a labor of love to be with both the patients and the students on their intersecting journeys. They have been inspiring teachers and companions as I explored my own healing. The reciprocal giving and receiving has been its own reward. I hope *Medicine Hands* assists you on your journey. It is a privilege to be with you.

REFERENCES

1. Cancer Facts and Figures – 1998. American Cancer Society. 1998.

2. Singh, U. P. Yogic Massage in Treating Stress and Other Conditions. *Massage Therapy Journal.* 1996;35(1):77-93.

3. Nicholson, G. L. The Metastatic Process of Cancer: Why Therapy Can Fail. *Your Patient and Cancer.* Winter 1987. p. 25-31.

4. Pfeifer, K. Pathophysiology. In *Oncology Nursing.* St. Louis: Mosby-Year Book, Inc., 1997.

5. White, J. An Interview with Sue Carlson. *Oregon AMTA Newsletter.* Summer 1997.

- *By the age of 75, Australian men have a one in three lifetime risk of having cancer; women have a one in four risk.*

- *It is estimated that one in three Britons are at risk of developing cancer at some point in their lives.*

- *Forty percent of Canadian men and 35 percent of women are at risk of developing cancer.*

Sources:

Giles, G.; K. Whitfield; V. Thursfield; and M. Staples. *Canstat: Cancer in Victoria*. Anti-Cancer Council of Victoria. 1997.

The Challenge We Face: The Latest Cancer Statistics. Cancer Research Campaign. 1997.

Canadian Cancer Statistics 1998. National Cancer Institute of Canada. 1998.

Chapter 2

Dispelling the Myths About Metastasis:

Facts About How Cancer Spreads

How cancer develops and progresses is still only partially known. However, it is safe to draw some conclusions regarding bodywork and metastasis. The more the medical profession understands how cancer spreads, the more apparent it is that previous fears about massaging people with cancer are unfounded. The concern that increasing the circulation will cause cancer cells to release from the primary tumor and spread to distant sites is an old wives' tale based on incomplete information. This attitude is understandable in light of prior knowledge. Until the 1970's, it was thought that the ability of tumors to invade or spread to distant sites was the result of simple growth pressure as the tumorous mass increased in size. This alone does not explain how cancer cells travel to secondary sites, nor why certain tumors can grow to a significant size, exert considerable pressure, but never

Benzo[a]pyrene causes cancer in a simple, direct way. Nearly all living things have in common a group of cellular enzymes responsible for detoxifying and metabolizing possibly harmful chemical invaders. When this enzyme group encounters benzo[a]pyrene, it inserts oxygen into the foreign molecule, the first step toward breaking it down. However, in a strange twist of fate, this addition activates benzo[a]pyrene rather than detoxifies it. The altered molecule now has the ability to bond tightly to a strand of DNA — that is, to one of the cell's chromosomes along which lie the organism's genes. A chemical invader so attached is called a DNA adduct, and it has the power to alter the structure of the DNA strand and produce a genetic mutation. If uncorrected, this type of damage can become a crucial step leading to the formation of cancer.

— SANDRA STEINGRABER,
Living Downstream

invade or metastasize. Research has shown that pressure alone is not sufficient to cause a tumor to become invasive.[1]

Scientists now know that accumulated genetic mutations are the primary reasons for normal cells to be transformed into tumor cells. These changes are responsible for uncontrolled cell growth and the ability of cancer cells to invade and spread to distant sites.[1] Approximately ten percent of defective genes are inherited, while the rest are acquired over the course of a lifetime. Many of the acquired mutations happen as a result of environmental factors. Through the years the strands of DNA that compose genes can be damaged by carcinogens such as smoke, pesticides, UV rays, diet, chemicals produced by the body, or microbes such as viruses, bacteria, or parasites. Genetic damage is also acquired because cells naturally make mistakes in the copying of DNA even without the influence of environmental agents. No matter what the origins of genetic injury, if the mutations occur in the growth-controlling genes the cell is given misinformation about how it should reproduce. Eventually this can result in tumors, some of which will be benign while others will become cancerous.[2]

So far, three classes of genes that play a major role in the development of cancer have been uncovered. The first group, oncogenes, cause excessive cell proliferation when mutation occurs. The second class, tumor suppressor genes, normally stifle tumor growth by acting as a braking system that halts inappropriate growth. When they are inactivated by mutations, uncontrolled cell proliferation is allowed to go unchecked.[2] Injured DNA repair genes are the third major category known to be involved in tumor growth. These genes "help to check and maintain the integrity of DNA, which is often damaged during replication. Without these mechanisms, the chances that a damaged gene will be repaired" are lowered, increasing the chance that the damage will be permanently transmitted to descendant cells.[3]

Cancer doesn't happen over night. In most cases, neoplasms have their beginnings decades before patients present to their physician with a palpable tumor or with symptoms associated with an established cancer such as severe fatigue or blood in the stool.[2,4] By the time of the treatment, approximately 60 percent of patients with solid tumors already have metastases or micrometastases.[5]

Initially, a neoplasm begins when a normal cell mutates, increasing its "propensity to proliferate when it would normally rest."[2] These transformed cells look normal, but they reproduce at a higher than usual rate. Years later, one in a million of these hyperplastic cells may be affected by another genetic mutation, causing further malfunctions in cell growth. At this stage, cells not only continue the excess growth, but the descendants take on an abnormal shape and orientation. This tissue is said to be dysplasic. After a time, if another mutation damages the cell's DNA, the growth and appearance become even more abnormal. At this point the neoplasm is still contained within the boundaries of the original tissue, and may remain so indefinitely, or not. It is not yet understood why certain masses remain localized and others become aggressively malignant. Researchers believe that tumors are propelled toward invasiveness by another accumulation of genetic transformations.[2]

The upcoming sections will indicate the complexity of metastatic development, an internal event directed by genetic forces. Massage in no way influences the rise of genetic mutations responsible for cancer and can be safely administered with proper modifications.

QUALITIES OF CANCER CELLS

As a result of genetic mutations, tumor cells acquire many qualities that cause them to function much differently than normal cells. Normal cells conduct themselves in an orderly manner, adhering to one another, stopping growth when contact is made with another cell, dividing only when attached to an anchor point. Tumor cells, on the other hand, are rowdy renegades in which the inhibition mechanisms have failed. They grow and divide, crowding the space they occupy, until the cells are piled on each other in an unorganized mass.[6]

Another quality of malignant cells that is responsible for their ability to spread is a lack of adhesiveness due to low levels of fibronectin on the cell surface. Fibronectin is a major element in the formation of the matrix in which all cells are embedded and which anchors cells in place within the tissues; it also serves as an organizing grid for the integral proteins of the cell surface. The lack of it allows cancer cells to effortlessly slip away from the parental mass. Not only do cancer cells lack adhesiveness, these aberrant cells are "anchorage independent" and can divide while suspended in a liquid medium.[6] When normal cells are denied anchorage, they stop reproducing and commit "cellular suicide," thereby safeguarding the integrity of tissues.[7]

Tumor cells are able to accomplish their feats on only a fraction of the growth factors normal cells would require. Some cancer cells even grow in the absence of these factors, which would seem to indicate that they make their own growth factors. In addition, metastatic cells are highly permeable, which means they can transport materials such as glucose and amino acids across the cell membrane at a rate higher than normal cells.[6]

The lining of body cavities, blood and lymphatic vessels, the outer part of the skin, interiors of the respiratory and digestive tracts, and glandular tissue are made of epithelial cells. These cells are designed to protect the body's underlying tissues, or in the case of glandular epithelium, constitute the secreting portion of glands.[8] This layer of cells forms a barrier that most normal cells cannot breach.[7] However, invading tumor cells have the ability to secrete enzymes (collagenases) that degrade the basement membrane and other extracellular matrices, allowing the cells to digest their way

CANCER
deep, angry red
yearning
burning
twisting
turning
eating bones and flesh
screaming to be heard
without uttering a word

— Dana Doolin-Frank, L.M.T.

through surrounding tissue.[6,7,9,10] (Figure 2-1) This ability to penetrate the epithelial basement membrane and enter the underlying interstitial stroma, allows them to gain access to lymphatics and blood vessels.[6,11] This is a major difference between invasive and non-invasive tumors.[6,10,11] The loss of the basement membrane correlates with an increased incidence of metastases.[4] In normal cells, enzymes are produced that inhibit these collagenases, but in metastatic cells not enough inhibitor is produced to neutralize the production of collagenase, creating an imbalance. This degradation, or injury to the surrounding tissues, causes the normal tissue to respond to the injury by secreting growth factors, which the metastatic cells take advantage of to continue proliferating.[9]

Tumor cells that possess the ability to induce new capillary growth, or neovascularization, are much more apt to spread. Most likely, neovascularization, also known as angiogenesis, is the result of mutated tumor cells. Without a blood supply to provide the needed nutrients, neoplasms cannot grow more than a few millimeters. Tumors that lack this ability remain in situ, a steady state in which the number of new cells equals the number of dying cells. For unknown reasons, an in situ tumor can suddenly induce new capillary growth, allowing the mass to continue growing and invade adjacent tissue. "Once neovascularization occurs, hundreds of new capillaries converge on the tiny tumor; each vessel soon has a thick coat of rapidly dividing tumor cells."[12] Within months the tumor may grow to a cubic centimeter, containing about one billion tumor cells. To make matters worse, the endothelial cells of the new capillaries release different proteins that can stimulate proliferation or cell motility, increasing the likelihood that cancer cells will leave the primary tumor and migrate into the bloodstream. The development of new capillaries is an important component of the metastatic process; by the time a tumor is large enough to detect, angiogenesis is usually well underway.[12]

It is these qualities of uncontrolled proliferation, lack of adhesiveness, anchorage independence, diminished need for growth factors, and the ability to secrete degradative enzymes and induce new capillary growth that are associated with the ability of tumor cells to spread. The spreading occurs irrespective of patients' activities. It happens while watching TV, cooking dinner, playing with the children, or even sleeping. Avoiding massage will not stop these rogue cells from slipping away from the original tumor. This is not to say that bodyworkers are free to work without considering the location of tumors and other factors. As shall be seen later, there are reasons for adjusting the sessions a cancer patient receives.

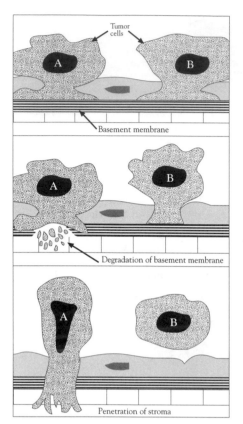

Figure 2-1. The Use of Degradative Enzymes

After a metastatic tumor cell adheres to the endothelium and penetrates to the subendothelial basement membrane, it releases enzymes that degrade elements of the basement membrane. (Cell A) Cells that cannot degrade the extra-cellular matrix cannot invade the organ and eventually move on to another site or die in the bloodstream. (Cell B)[10]

THE SPREAD OF CANCER

The spread of cancer is not a random event, it is a "logical, coordinated process."[5] Malignant cells spread from the primary tumor by two major processes: direct spreading to adjoining areas or metastatic spread to distant areas. The dissemination may be by one or both processes, since spread via one route may create access to the other.[5]

DIRECT SPREAD

Direct spread, the penetration and destruction of adjacent tissue, is the result of many factors. Local invasion is enhanced by the ability of malignant cells to stimulate new capillary formation which greatly increases the tumor's growth rate. This rapid proliferation produces densely packed, expanding masses of cells that exert pressure on adjacent tissues, forcing fingerlike projections into neighboring areas. Tumors then spread along natural fracture lines into spaces that separate in response to pressure, such as interstitial or cerebrospinal spaces or the abdominal cavity.[1,5,6,7]

Malignant cells may also invade by secreting enzymes that break down the basement membrane of tissues, resulting in the penetration of body cavities. After spreading into neighboring areas and penetrating body cavities, such as the pleural and peritoneal cavities, cancer cells can attach to the surfaces within the cavity.[5]

Initially, local invasion happens as direct tumor extension. However, at some point, because of a lack of adhesiveness between cells as well as their increased motility, cells or clumps of cells detach from the parental mass. Although mechanical force may influence the invasion process, it is not the primary cause and is insufficient to bring about metastasis on its own. Bodyworkers, however, should be mindful of tumor sites, because additional force on the tumor may contribute to the pressure already taking place due to uncontrolled growth of the neoplasm. Fortunately, even if a malignant cell releases from the primary site, the formation of a secondary tumor is not an automatic outcome. A malignant cell must possess the ability to erode, invade, and pass through the local stromal layer in order to continue the metastatic sequence.[1]

METASTATIC SPREAD

Once a tumor cell has left the parental mass, it must successfully complete a series of steps to establish a metastatic lesion. The inability to complete each of the steps will stop the metastatic cascade. A tumor cell must be able to invade the blood system or lymph vessels, travel in the circulatory system to the distant site, arrest in a congenial site, adhere to the endothelial lining, reinvade the distant organ or tissue, and establish a new blood supply.[7] Despite their many capabilities, it is so difficult for the migrating cells to complete all of these requirements that very few manage to colonize a distant site.

LYMPHATIC DISSEMINATION

The spread to nonadjacent sites occurs via two entryways, lymphatic channels or blood vessels. Often, because the vascular and lymphatic systems are interconnected, both are involved.[1,5] For many types of cancer the first evidence of spreading is a mass in the lymph nodes that drain the area where the primary tumor is located.[5] The spread of malignant cells into the lymph nodes is a significant occurrence, as lymph nodes are involved in about half of all fatal cancers. Once malignant cells lodge in lymph nodes they have several possible fates: 1) die of a local inflammatory reaction; 2) wither and die because of a lack of the proper environment; 3) remain dormant; 4) grow into a mass.[5,13]

At one time the filtering action of the lymph nodes was believed to be the cause of nodal metastasis. Research, however, has shown filtration to be only a minor influence. Most likely the interaction between physiochemical changes on the cancer cell's surface and the lymph node determines whether and where cancer cells will lodge in the lymphatic system. Logically, it might follow that the lymph nodes that drain the primary tumors would test positive before more distant nodes. And while this sometimes can be the case, other metastatic cells bypass local lymph nodes and settle in distant ones, indicating that other influences are at work. Just as blood-borne metastases are not random or completely the result of anatomical flow routes, neither are nodal metastases. Most likely site specific recognition plays a part in the location of these neoplasms.[5]

For cancer patients with lymphatic involvement there is confusion within the bodywork community about which touch modalities to perform. Many oncologists fail to see how comfort-oriented massage would contribute to the spread of cancer. Lymphatic circulation occurs naturally as a result of skeletal muscles contracting, which compresses lymph vessels and forces the movement of lymph. Gentle massage does not increase lymphatic circulation any more than the activities of daily life such as exercising, shopping, or caring for children, activities which doctors urge their patients to engage in.

Modalities with the specific intent of stimulating lymphatic movement, such as Manual Lymphatic Drainage, officially advise that their techniques are contraindicated for people with active cancer. A statement made in the 1995 consensus document issued by the Executive Committee of the International Society of Lymphology concerning the use of manual lymphedema treatment (MLT) for women with breast cancer may calm the doubts of lymphatic massage practitioners. "Rare reports suggest that MLT may promote metastatic disease, although theoretically only diffuse carcinomatous infiltrates [invasive cancer cells] which have already spread to lymph collectors as tumor emboli could be mobilized by mechanical compression. In these instances, the long-term prognosis for the patient is already poor, and some reduction of... swelling may be decidedly palliative. Mobilization of dormant tumor cells by arm compression in patients after treatment of carcinoma of the breast remains speculative and thus far unconvincing and unfounded."[14]

Vocabulary

Avascular

Lacking in blood vessels.

DNA

A nucleic acid that forms two long, twisting chains which are found on the chromosomes and carry genetic information.

Emboli

A detached mass of cells in the bloodstream that may consist of bits of tissue, tumor cells, fat globules, air bubbles, clumps of bacteria, and foreign bodies.

Endothelial

A form of squamous cell that lines the blood and lymphatic vessels, the heart, and various other body cavities.

Enzymes

Substances that affect the speed of chemical changes, a catalyst.

Source: Thomas C.L., ed. *Taber's Cyclopedic Medical Dictionary*. Philadelphia: F.A. Davis Co. 1993.

HEMATOGENOUS SPREAD (BLOOD-BORNE)

While the local spread of cancer occurs predominately through the lymphatic vessels, spreading to remote organs and tissues is almost always via the bloodstream. One of the capacities of invasive tumors is the ability to create its own blood supply. Once neovascularization occurs within the primary tumor, cancer cells can be released into the circulatory system. The basement membranes of these newly formed vessels are porous, which may explain how tumor cells enter the bloodstream from a vascularized tumor.[1,5] Tumor cells also can pass into veins via the lymphatic-venous connection or by directly invading veins and capillaries.[5,11] However, the presence of tumor cells in the blood does not mean that metastasis is a foregone conclusion. Because of a lack of adhesiveness between cell surfaces, vascularized tumors continually shed cancer cells as they increase in size.[1] Even though a large number of cancer cells may be in the patient's circulatory system, the chance of successful metastasis is low. It is estimated that fewer than one in 10,000 cancer cells that enter the bloodstream lives to reach another organ. Even fewer successfully implant themselves. At every step they must escape the many controls that keep normal cells in place.[1,7,10,11,15,16]

Cancer cells face many threats while in the circulatory system, such as the mechanical force of blood turbulence. Hemodynamics has been suggested as a possible factor in that vascular pressure and flow rate may be too high in certain areas like skin and skeletal muscles to allow cancer cells to come to rest there.[13] Apparently, the longer cancer cells remain in the circulatory system, the higher their death rate. Inhibiting the coagulation process also seems to keep cancer cells circulating longer and decreases the number of tumor emboli that arrest in vascular beds.[5]

On the other hand, constituents of the blood system can assist the metastatic process. Tumor cells sometimes adhere to blood cells, such as leukocytes, lymphocytes, and platelets, as well as fibrin and other tumor cells.[1,5,7] Platelets, which produce their own growth factors, may help cancer cells survive in the blood.[7] Adhering to these other cells helps protect the tumor cells from circulating immune cells and produces enlarged emboli, increasing the likelihood they will arrest in capillaries or in the target organ.[4,7]

It is hypothesized that some metastatic deposits can be predicted from the blood flow route. The most frequent site of arrest in many cancer cell types is the first capillary bed encountered.[1,7] This might account for the higher number of lung tumors, as the lung is the first site the shed cells encounter after the venous circulation. However, even when metastasis occurs in the first organ encountered, site specific recognition most likely plays a part.[1,7,10] Studies show that clusters of tumor cells do not always come to rest in the first capillary bed they enter, but are able to pass through capillaries, even capillaries smaller in size.[7] Even though blood flow routes may contribute to the process, evidence shows that on its own, the trapping of cells is generally not sufficient to promote the formation of metastatic colonies.[7,10]

Vocabulary

Hemodynamics
The forces involved in circulating blood through the body.

Hyperplastic
Excessive growth of normal cells in the normal tissue arrangement of an organ.

Interstitial
Spaces within an organ or tissue including the space between cells.

Motility
The ability to move.

Stroma
The foundation supporting tissues of an organ.

Source: Thomas C.L., ed. *Taber's Cyclopedic Medical Dictionary*. Philadelphia: F.A. Davis Co. 1993.

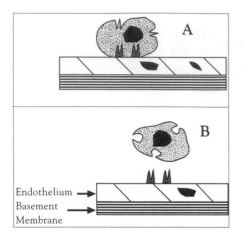

Figure 2-2 Site specific cell adhesion

Tumor cells that adhere to certain sites do so in part because they possess receptors for those organs. (Panel A) Tumor cells that lack receptors for a specific organ will fail to bind and pass through the organ vasculature into the collecting veins (Panel B).

Tumor cell arrests frequently are dependent upon a match between the tumor and organ or tissue. This hypothesis is known as the seed and soil theory. It suggests that certain organs and tissues possess special characteristics (soil) that enable cancer cells (seeds) to flourish.[4,11,15] Perhaps a characteristic that might make the soil of an organ congenial to tumor growth is the presence of specific growth factors found at those sites.[10] Other evidence points toward an idea of adhesive-specificity, where particular cancers bind to certain types of tissue. Studies of blood-borne implantation have found that instead of traveling haphazardly through the circulatory system, the cells home in to certain sites. In part, this happens because they contain adhesion molecules that recognize the "molecular address system"[7] to the surfaces of certain tissues or organs.[1,7,9] (Figure 2-2) Migration to these sites appears to be under the influence of chemotactic factors (attraction and repulsion to a chemical stimulus) which influence the tumor cells to travel in the direction of certain growth factors rather than moving about in hit-or-miss fashion.[1,17] A combination of mechanisms is probably responsible for determining where tumor cells arrest: adhesive properties, chemotaxis, and responses to growth factors present in different organs and tissues.[4,10,11] Some researchers have put forward the idea that the preference for certain metastatic sites may be genetically determined.[1,17]

After the tumor cell emboli has arrested a number of things must happen in order for the sequence to continue. It must adhere to the blood vessel's endothelial lining, and then invade that wall to pass through to the basement membrane surrounding the tissue or organ. Then the tumor cells must invade that protective wall with degradative enzymes. This happens either directly through thin-walled capillaries, or by producing enzymes that degrade the basement membrane. In turn, this damage to tissue creates an inflammatory response, leading to further release of degradative enzymes which facilitate tumor cell invasion through the capillary beds.[4]

A number of things can happen once cancer cells reinvade remote tissue. They may die, or lie dormant for years and then grow to a large size long after the primary tumor has been removed, or they may begin growing to a large size immediately. In order to create a new tumor, the attacking cells must have the ability to establish their own blood supply.[12]

It is not known what causes metastatic tumor cells to remain in a dormant stage, or what causes them to eventually become active. Possibly small populations of tumor cells remain in an avascular phase for prolonged periods, which may explain dormant metastases to some degree. It is not unheard of in breast cancer for metastases to appear in the vertebrae 30 years later. It also not unusual for the metastatic growth to show itself before the primary tumor. A patient may present with a broken bone and then be found to have a primary carcinoma of the thyroid that has metastasized to the bone; or a skin metastases may be the first symptom of latent gastric cancer.[5,13]

HOST FACTORS

The way in which tumors of the same type and grade metastasize varies from one person to the next. This has led some researchers to conclude that factors related to the host contribute to metastatic potential. These factors include genetics, which was covered in the opening of the chapter, the immune system, age, hormones, and trauma.[4]

While the immune system does not appear to play a part in the genetic transformations that initiate cell proliferation, there is evidence that the health of a person's immune system influences whether and how cancer will develop. Many researchers believe that cancer cells are continually being created in our bodies, and then destroyed by such defenses as macrophages and natural killer cells.[5] These immune cells may even play a role in eliminating micrometastases.[1] However, when the "surveillance system" breaks down, malignancies occur.[18]

Research has shown certain cancer cells that normally wouldn't metastasize will do so in experimental animals whose immune systems are suppressed. There also is evidence of increased occurrence and virulence of cancer in people who are immuno-suppressed, suggesting that some tumors develop and spread more easily when immune function is abnormal.[1] Massage research, particularly that of Tiffany Field and her colleagues, is showing a positive relationship between massage and the immune system.[19] Perhaps bodywork will eventually be proven to have an inhibitory effect on the development of cancer.

Certain functions of the immune system, however, can help establish metastatic disease.[1,20] One of these functions, which is relevant to bodywork, is the immune response caused by injury to tissue. Just as enlarging tumors trigger the inflammatory response by damaging neighboring tissue, deep massage, too, can induce this reaction. Both events cause inflammatory cells to produce enzymes that degrade the basement membrane of surrounding tissue as well as blood vessels, thereby facilitating tumor cell invasion. In addition, vasodilation occurs, causing increased permeability of blood vessels. Tumor cells are further aided by combining with elements of the immune system that accumulate in the area, such as leukocytes and macrophages, as well as constituents present in the clotting process, such as platelets and fibrin, to form emboli. The likelihood of cancer cells arresting in a capillary bed is increased by this process. In light of the above knowledge, it is inadvisable for people with metastatic disease to receive deep, traumatic massage to any part of the body.

Another determinant in the development of cancer is the age of the host. In studies with animals, older animals have been shown to be less susceptible to metastasis than younger ones.[13] Perhaps this has to do with the greater level of growth factors present in the young. On the other hand, statistics for people show age contributes greatly in the development of tumors. Between the ages of 40 and 59,

American women have a one in 11 chance of being diagnosed with cancer. That number increases dramatically to one in five women ages 60 to 79.[21]

Certain types of tumors appear to increase, regress, or arrest because of hormones. One example of the relationship between a hormone and tumors is that of estrogen to endometrial cancer. Studies have shown that menopausal women who take replacement estrogen have an increased incidence of endometrial cancer.[22] Another example is glucocortocoids, a group of hormones secreted from the adrenal glands. High levels of these substances have been implicated in the growth of tumors. Elevated amounts of glucocortocoids can be caused by physical and emotional stress.[23]

In the final chapter of her doctoral thesis, "The Effect of Therapeutic Massage on Post Surgical Outcomes," Martha Brown Menard posits that "massage may actually have a protective effect against tumor growth." Because high levels of glucocortocoids, including cortisol, have been connected with tumor growth. interventions known to lower elevated cortisol levels may have an inhibitory effect on tumor growth. Cortisol levels, a yardstick commonly used in research to measure physical and psychological stress, consistently have been shown to decrease as a result of massage.[23]

Recent trauma, such as incisions, laser-induced injury, or electrocautery (to cauterize with an electrically heated wire) seems to predispose a particular site to implantation by malignant cells. Animal studies have shown that tumor cells injected into acutely traumatized tissue will implant and grow, whereas cells injected into the same untraumatized tissue will not. The time interval between trauma and injection of cancer cells is important. The nearer the time of trauma, the greater the incidence of metastasis, which may have to do with factors related to blood clotting. Cancer cells form emboli by attaching to platelet cells, which are major components in the blood clotting process.[11] The key to this occurrence is "implantation by malignant cells." It is highly unlikely that benign cells implanted in the same way would proliferate. However, it is important that massage therapists pay close attention to this information as it supports the idea of giving gentle massage and avoiding deep pressure that may cause trauma to the body.

Some doctors have wondered whether cancer cells are jarred loose during the trauma of manipulation or surgical incision causing dissemination via vascular and lymphatic channels.[7,13] No research has been performed to answer this question. Just in case, surgeons take care in handling and manipulating tumors during resection (the cutting off or out of a portion of a structure).[13] Bodyworkers, too, should take care and avoid massaging areas known to have a tumor, as it may influence the metastatic potential.[5,13] But as Bernie Siegel points out, there is more to a person than their tumor.[24] For instance, someone with breast cancer could still have their legs, feet, arms, hands, back, and neck massaged.

A Summary of Bodywork Implications

After an examination of the metastatic process, there are apparent implications with regard to bodywork:

- It is not possible to know at any given time whether any client is cancer free. There are always aberrant cells present in the body, or cancer cells can lie dormant and then years later become active. Despite following intake protocols to the letter, many bodyworkers have unknowingly massaged someone with cancer. Patients often times do not present to their physician until a tumor is well established, and by the time of the initial diagnosis, a high percentage already have metastases. However, practitioners have acted in a judicious manner if they followed accepted intake procedures, took a written health history, and obtained physician approval for clients whose medical condition warranted it. When a massage client has been diagnosed with cancer, at least the therapist is cognizant of the situation and can adjust the sessions accordingly.

- Cancer spreads even while patients are involved in completely sedate activities such as sitting or sleeping, consequently, gentle massage can be given to areas of the body not affected by cancer.

- Massaging the site of a tumor is contraindicated, as the mechanical force on the tumor may contribute to the pressure build-up already taking place by the uncontrolled growth of the neoplasm. Although mechanical pressure is not the primary cause of invasiveness, it may be influential.

- Deep traumatic massage to any part of the body is inadvisable for those with active cancer. As will be seen in later chapters, people with cancer can bruise more easily due to chemotherapy, radiation, and medications. Injury to tissues causes the immune response to be activated. This process can facilitate embolization as well as produce enzymes that degrade surrounding tissue, both of which are factors in metastasis.

- Bodyworkers wishing to perform lymph drainage techniques should speak to the lymphoma patient's physician.

Final Thoughts

A fellow bodyworker recounted a story about a woman with lymphoma who came to her with a doctor's order for massage. The massage therapist, however, told the woman she would not work with her because massage increased lymphatic flow, which would speed up the flow of cancer cells in the lymph.

I have treated many, many cancer patients using CranioSacral Therapy and SomatoEmotional Release over about a 25 year period. I have yet to see anything that arouses the slightest suspicion in me that any of this work contributes to metastases. I have seen it do a lot of good however, even complete remission in some cases. Further, I do not believe that massage contributes to metastasis unless it is very deep, traumatic massage.

— Dr. John Upledger, D.O. originator of CranioSacral Therapy

The massage therapist explained to the client that she didn't want to be responsible for contributing to her cancer. The woman pleaded with the practitioner, saying that she was certain massage would help. When the bodyworker called the client's doctor he urged her to proceed with the session. He supported the idea that the patient's belief in the potential of massage was important and could bring about a positive outcome. The physician also went on to explain that the spread of cancer is not brought about by speeding up lymphatic flow, but is dependent on the metastatic potential of the tumor cells.

Metastatic potential, like the initial growth of tumor cells, is heavily dependent on genetic factors that are either inherited or acquired. Acquired influences occur when sufficient genetic mutations have accumulated, usually over decades, as a result of DNA being damaged by carcinogenic agents or by naturally occurring errors in the replication of DNA. Many of the exact genetic defects responsible for the rise of tumorous masses are known to researchers, and it is only a matter time before the roots of metastasis are also traced to the mutations of specific genes, not to an increase in circulation. Cancer cells are able to invade the blood and lymphatic systems, travel to a distant site, and establish a new blood supply, because they are receiving misinformation from malfunctioning genes. If increased circulation caused tumor cells to spread more rapidly, physical therapists would not carry out vigorous exercise with people who have cancer, respiratory therapists would not perform percussion the backs of post-surgical patients, and doctors would not allow patients to jog, swim, or play in the World Series, as Eric Davis of the Baltimore Orioles did in 1997 while undergoing chemotherapy.

There is no evidence to suggest that touch or gentle massage causes metastasis, but there is proof that it greatly benefits many cancer patients, both physically and emotionally. The data has shown light massage to positively affect symptoms related to cancer or side effects from treatment regimens, such as nausea, fatigue, insomnia, and pain. Patients report an increased sense of well-being, with reduction in anxiety and the sense of isolation, as well as increased relaxation and decreased muscle tension. As *Medicine Hands* proceeds, it will become apparent that care, caution, and a soft touch are the watch words when massaging people with cancer, not fear. This is not to say that metastasis is a trivial matter. It is a very serious one. Bodywork, however, can be adapted to insure that it is beneficial to people with cancer.

REFERENCES

1. Soltis, M.J.; S.M. Hubbard; and E.C. Kohn. The Biology of Invasion and Metastases in *Cancer Nursing: A Comprehensive Textbook*. Philadelphia: W.B. Saunders, 1996.

2. Weinberg, R.A. How Cancer Arises. *Scientific American*. 1996; 275(3):62-70.

3. Oliff, A.; J.B. Gibbs; and F. McCormick. New Molecular Targets for Cancer Therapy. *Scientific American*. 1996; 275(3):144-149.

4. Groenwald, S.L. Invasion and Metastasis in *Cancer Nursing: Principles and Practices*. Boston: Jones and Bartlett, 1993.

5. Pfeifer, K.A. Pathophysiology in *Oncology Nursing*. St. Louis: Mosby-Year Book, 1997.

6. Groenwald, S.L. Differences Between Normal and Cancer Cells in *Cancer Nursing: Principles and Practices*. Boston: Jones and Bartlett, 1993.

7. Ruoslahti, E. How Cancer Spreads. *Scientific American*. 1996; 275(3):72-77.

8. Tortora, G. *Introduction to the Human Body*. Menlo Park: Addison Wesley Longman, 1997.

9. Brylawski, R. Unraveling the Mystery of Metastasis. *Oncology Times*. February, 1991: p. 3.

10. Zetter, B.R. The Cellular Basis of Site-Specific Tumor Metastasis. *Seminars in Medicine of the Beth Israel Hospital*. Boston. 1990; 322(9):605-611.

11. Scanlon, E.F. and S. Murthy. Basic Science Overview – The Process of Metastasis. *CA – A Cancer Journal for Clinicians*. 1991;41(5):301-305.

12. Folkman, J. Fighting Cancer by Attacking its Blood Supply. *Scientific American*. 1996; 275(3):150-154.

13. Kupchella, C.E. and R.M. Burton. Cellular Biology of Cancer in *Cancer Nursing: Principles and Practices*. Boston: Jones and Bartlett, 1987.

14. The Diagnosis and Treatment of Peripheral Lymphedema: Consensus Document of the International Society of Lymphology Executive Committee. *Lymphology*. 1995; 28:113-117.

15. Killion, J.J. and I.J. Fidler. The Biology of Tumor Metastasis. *Seminars in Oncology*. 1989; 16(2): 106-115.

16. Nicholson, G.L. The Metastatic Process of Cancer: Why Therapy Can Fail. *Your Patient and Cancer.* p. 25-31, Winter 1987.

17. Templeton, D.J. and R.A. Weinberg. *Principles of Cancer Biology in American Cancer Society Textbook of Clinical Oncology.* Atlanta: American Cancer Society, 1995.

18. Nuland, S. *How We Die.* New York: Knopf, 1994.

19. Ironson, G.; T. Field; F. Scalfidi; M. Hashimoto; et al. Massage Therapy is Associated with Enhancement of the Immune System's Cytotoxic Capacity. *International Journal of Neuroscience.* 1996; 84:205-217.

20. Braun, D.P. and S.L. Groenwald. Relation of the Immune System to Cancer in *Cancer Nursing: Principles and Practices.* Boston: Jones and Bartlett, 1993.

21. *Cancer Facts and Figures – 1998.* American Cancer Society. 1998.

22. Yarbro, J.W. Milestones in Our Understanding of the Causes of Cancer in *Cancer Nursing: Principles and Practices.* Boston: Jones and Bartlett, 1993.

23. Menard, M.B. The Effect of Therapeutic Massage on Post Surgical Outcomes. Doctoral Thesis. University of Virginia. 1995.

24. Siegel, B. Letter to the Editor. *Massage Therapy Journal.* 1996;35(2):12.

Chapter 3

Touch—Rx for Body, Mind, and Heart:

A Review of the Research and Literature

I f a drug were discovered that provided the many benefits massage gives to cancer patients, pharmaceutical companies would be falling all over themselves and each other to bottle it. And, if oncologists understood its value, they would write as many prescriptions for massage as for analgesics. One of the marvels of skilled, attentive touch is that it can relieve discomfort on every level. Although the data is still scarce in most areas, what does exist shows that bodywork could be prescribed in conjunction with other interventions for many of the physical discomforts of cancer and its treatment, such as insomnia, nausea, fatigue, and muscular tension; for emotional distresses such as anxiety, depression, and loneliness; or for improving mental factors, such as concentration and self-image. Granted, pharmacological interventions are absolutely necessary, but percodan cannot touch the pain in the soul, and prednisone can't heal wounded emotions.

... human touch can communicate the energy of life itself.
— WILLIAM FRICK

Research into the use of bodywork for cancer patients is sparse and still in its infancy. Published studies have had small patient numbers and lack the rigor demanded by the medical community, but several projects are underway that meet the accepted standards of research. The data collected to this point and the anecdotal evidence show that various bodywork modalities are efficacious in relieving a host of cancer's maladies, both physical and emotional. Improvement has been reported for symptoms such as nausea, fatigue, muscular tension, pain, lymphedema, isolation, and anxiety. However, it is important to emphasize that bodywork, like other relaxation therapies, cannot replace standard pain medication, but should be viewed as one strategy within a multifaceted treatment plan.

MASSAGE – A THERAPY FOR THE WHOLE PERSON

Oncology is at the forefront in medicine in its treatment of the whole person. Often, cancer care centers provide a menu of varied adjuvant therapies such as visualization techniques, art therapy, and support groups. Massage too has a role to play along with these treatments and would help in creating cancer care that is even more comprehensive. Bodywork is unique in its ability to simultaneously provide healing in many areas of the patient's life. Skilled touch can increase quality of life, lend emotional support, and decrease pain and other physical discomforts.

PAIN

Pain is the sensation of extreme discomfort, and suffering is the 'story', or our feelings toward it.

*— JOAN HALIFAX,
Founder of the Project on Being with Dying*

Pain is one of the most feared elements of the cancer experience, and something that affects patients' comfort and quality of life. Kathleen Foley, Chief of Pain Service at Memorial Sloan-Kettering Cancer Center, believes that not only is providing pain relief essential in and of itself, but it also can improve the patient's chances of survival. "Pain can erode a patient's willingness to continue treatment, even to live."[1] Severe pain not only affects the will to live or response to treatment,[2,3] it may hinder the healing process, or prolong hospitalization.[4]

At best, the management of pain is a complex and inexact science.[4] Despite advances in pain medications, cancer pain or discomfort related to treatment cannot always be completely managed through analgesics. Dr. David Weissman, associate professor of oncology and hematology (blood diseases) at the Medical College of Wisconsin, estimates that 50-75 percent of cancer pain is inadequately treated in the U.S.[5] The research of Dorrepaal[6] et al put the percentage at 50, while patients in a study done by Daut[2] et al reported that pain treatments or medications provide only 68 percent relief. Partially this is due to limitations of the drugs, but it is also a consequence of misconceptions by physicians who underprescribe medication for fear of patients developing drug tolerance or addiction. This fear, however, is unwarranted, as numerous studies indicate that cancer patients rarely develop psychological dependence on narcotics.[6]

Combining relaxation techniques, such as massage, with standard pain medications may help to address the issue of inadequately treated pain. Several studies that looked at the use of Swedish Massage with cancer patients indicate that technique to be beneficial in decreasing some patients' cancer pain. Twenty-two percent of those in Tope's study mentioned that their massages assisted in symptom management, which included pain[7]; subjects in the study by Ferrell-Tory and Glick reported a 60 percent reduction in perceived pain[8]; while one-third of the patients cited a reduction in pain in Wilkinson's study.[9] Weinrich and Weinrich found that the male cancer patients in their project had significantly less pain following a ten minute massage, but the female patients reported no significant decrease.[10] Menard's study of female surgical patients indicated a trend toward decreased pain as well as the use of less pain medication as a result of daily massages during hospitalization.[11] Her research may shed light on what had previously only been anecdotal evidence, that massage may enhance the effectiveness of pharmacological interventions.

Cancer pain is caused by a variety of influences, such as fear, beliefs based on prior experience, or physical influences such as bone or nerve compression. Because pain is the result of a multitude of forces, the ideal pain management program consists of a combination of drug and non-drug interventions.[2,3,12-15] When patients use a variety of pain reduction strategies, they perceive pain to be less intense.[3,15]

Two projects examined the use of a multi-modal pain reduction program that included massage. Nursing professor JoAnn Dalton studied 16 cancer patients who had disease-related pain (vs. treatment-related pain).[16] There were two experimental groups. Group A was taught only a relaxation strategy (progressive muscle relaxation), while Group B was taught the relaxation strategy plus distraction (music) and massage. Both groups were instructed to use these interventions whenever they felt pain while in the hospital and at home. Analgesics were never withheld from the experimental groups. Group C, the control group, received normal medical treatment only.

Group C showed the highest level of pain on the post-test, while both experimental groups reported a decrease in pain following the use of their respective interventions. No statistical significance

When you are lost in the black valley of pain, words grow frail and dumb. To be embraced and held warmly brings the only shelter and consolation.

— JOHN O'DONOHUE, ANAM CARA

Touch was never meant to be a luxury. It is a basic human need. It is an action that validates life and gives hope to both the receiver and the giver. The healing of touch is reciprocal.

— IRENE SMITH,
*co-founder of
Service through Touch*

existed in the amount of relief brought about by the two different experimental groups. Two of the subjects from Group B who used massage received no relief from that modality; however, the other three subjects reported "moderate" to "quite a lot of relief."

Diane Scott, nurse scientist at Memorial Sloan-Kettering Cancer Center, looked at the effect of a relaxation program that combined three different non-drug interventions on ten women who were receiving a highly nauseous chemotherapy regimen.[17] The relaxation protocol, given before and after chemo, consisted of slow stroke back massage given to the shoulders, neck, and back. During the massage patients were coached in a guided imagery technique and progressive relaxation.

The use of this technique resulted in a decrease in duration, frequency, and intensity of nausea and vomiting and a decrease in the volume of diarrhea. Patients' perception of the chemotherapy experience was improved compared to the known clinical response of patients receiving standard nursing support. The women reported less fear of the experience and a greater sense of control over their body. "Relaxation may help prevent... anticipatory nausea and vomiting and may support continued compliance with the difficult course of cancer treatment."

Despite the evidence that non-drug strategies such as relaxation training, biofeedback, massage, or hypnotherapy are useful in the treatment of pain, these techniques are seldom initiated by health care providers.[6,13] Chart audits in hospital settings show that as few as two percent of patients in pain received any type of non-drug intervention.[13] The emphasis in pain management is often on the technology. "Attempts are made to break the pain down into pieces, to find the right nerve to block, the right surgery, or the neurotransmitter that will explain or control the problem. But as much as any kind of illness, pain warrants a holistic approach to treatment."[4]

Pain control must be approached not only holistically, but must also be tailored to each individual. Just as no two people have pain in the same way,[3,4,14] no one protocol can be used universally for all patients. Finding the right combination of drugs, relaxation techniques, or positions is a matter of trial and error. Not only are each patient's pain needs unique, there is no way to predict which modalities will work best for them. One factor that could predict how well a particular strategy would work is the patient's expectations. Dalton found that subjects who had mild expectations reported mild relief, high expectations netted higher relief.

The severity of pain varies depending on the patient's perception of what is causing it. Groups that feel their pain is caused by the cancer or by something threatening are most at risk for settling into a sedentary life-style. Patients who believe their pain is the result of treatment tend to be more active, and those who feel their pain is caused by other factors, such as muscle tension, remain the most active. Twycross found that myofascial pain is the most common form of pain unrelated to cancer or treatment. Fascia is a tough connective tissue that covers every muscle, bone, nerve, artery, vein, and all of the internal organs. "Myo" is the root word for "muscle", so myofascial pain is pain related to the fascia covering muscles.

Lymphedema can also create pain when lymphatic obstruction occurs in the axilla, pelvis, or groin, causing a swollen limb.[12] When discomfort is caused by reasons unrelated to the disease or treatment, such as with myofascial pain, patients should be educated about these origins. It can be heartening to know that not every twinge is caused by the disease. This may put patients at ease and encourage them to remain active.[2,12]

Because the trend is toward shorter hospital stays, more of the care and management of pain is provided in the home by family members. Caring for cancer patients is difficult and complex enough for those with professional training, but for those who have not been prepared for such a role, the task can be overwhelming. Managing pain in the home setting is a major concern for patients and family caregivers. According to Ferrell, 70 percent of patients experience more pain at home, perhaps because they do not take their medications as prescribed.[14] Like doctors, family caregivers also fear drug addiction, tolerance, or respiratory depression, one of the side-effects of narcotics.[18] Many patients resist taking analgesics for fear their mind will be dulled or their bowels will become so sluggish that elimination is severely affected.

Teaching caregivers to administer the more benign methods of pain control may be a partial solution to the hesitancy family members have about giving analgesics. Because there is some anecdotal evidence that dosages can be reduced when used in combination with adjuvant pain therapies, caregivers could then give lesser amounts of narcotics. Caregivers instinctively, but often haphazardly, apply non-drug interventions such as re-positioning, touch, heat and cold, or relaxation techniques. While these strategies generally don't alleviate all pain, they are likely to be an effective component of the total pain-management program.[19]

In an overview of nonanalgesic approaches to pain control, Degner reported that relaxation therapy is the most frequently used technique. For some patients, traditional relaxation techniques such as progressive relaxation or guided imagery demand too much effort or are ineffective. Others simply don't like these approaches, and a few report that relaxation techniques actually increase their distress.[19] Massage might be more effective for those patients whose ability to concentrate is low or who prefer a more passive form of intervention.

Ferrell and Schneider's study of the "Experience and management of cancer pain at home," indicated that 60 percent of home patients used non-drug techniques to address pain. Massage was the second most commonly administered strategy. Foot massage was cited frequently, as well as general body massage.[14] Barbour et al. surveyed 58 cancer outpatients as to non-pharmacological methods they used to control pain. The four methods that provided the greatest relief were distraction, position change, massage, and heat.[20]

Most caregivers, however, have never received instruction from home health care staff about which strategies to employ in which situations. Often a method will be chosen that is inappropriate for the type of pain being experienced. If that therapy fails, the patient and caregiver will often abandon all other non-drug interventions as useless. It is important to view non-drug therapies as one part of a comprehensive pain management program and not as a replacement for medication. When patients receive inadequate analgesics, the non-pharmacological techniques tend to be ineffective, causing the family and patient to believe that "those things don't work."[13]

Rhiner et al. designed a three-part pain education program consisting of an overview of pain management, pharmacologic management of pain, and nondrug interventions.[13] In the nondrug portion of the educational program the patient had the opportunity to choose from a menu of five nondrug interventions: heat, cold, massage, relaxation/distraction, and imagery. Massage techniques included both hand massage and electric massage/vibration. The two most popular choices of non-pharmacological relief were heat and massage/vibration. Of the 40 patients, 70 percent selected heat and 63 percent chose massage/vibration. "Patients most often chose the vibration with heat, especially those patients with hip and leg pain." Perceived effectiveness was rated on a 0 to 4 scale (0, not at all effective to 4, very effective). Heat's effectiveness rating was 3.17, while massage's was 2.76. Interestingly, "distraction" (humorous or musical audio tapes) was rated as the most effective – 3.9. Patients were frequently reminded that the purpose of the nondrug methods was to enhance the effectiveness of the pharmacological interventions.

Family members often feel powerless to help when their loved one is in the throes of pain. Being able to effectively use non-pharmacological interventions may soothe the caregiver as much at the patient,[13] because when the patient is suffering, the family suffers too. Ferrell et al. put forward the idea of training caregivers to be "comfort coaches", much in the same way mothers have a birthing coach during delivery.[18]

QUALITY OF LIFE

More and more cancer is becoming a chronic illness, rather than just a terminal one. At one time the emphasis was on how long a patient lived with cancer, but now, quality of life has become equally important. For many cancer patients, pain, fatigue, and weakness interfere with their ability to perform daily functions and therefore with their quality of living.[2,3,6,12,14] In Arathuzik's study of 80 metastatic breast cancer patients, the main coping behavior when besieged by pain was withdrawal and inactivity. But research shows that when pain is effectively managed, patients remain more active and report fewer problems than those who give in to disability. Active patients generally have more energy and stamina which contributes to greater confidence, an ability to maintain independence, and can make the difference between "living" and "existing."[21]

Quality of life may even influence survival. One study of patients with metastatic breast cancer showed a correlation between these two elements.[22] Another study, reported by Justice, found that women who were depressed, apathetic, and fatigued following breast surgery for cancer had the "worst biologic status."[23] Depressed patients tend to use withdrawal to cope with pain, which sets off the cycle of inactivity and decreases peoples' quality of life.[3]

The topic of massage for depressed cancer patients has not been studied well enough to form definite conclusions, but the data is pointing toward a positive correlation. Thirty-five percent of Tope's massage subjects commented that their mood improved or they felt a greater sense of well being.Ferrell-Tory and Glick's subjects felt more relaxed and less anxious as a result of massage. Studies performed at the University of Miami School of Medicine's Touch Research Institute (TRI) may provide the best documentation of the use of massage for depression. Dr. Tiffany Fields and her colleagues at TRI have found massage to decrease depression in teenage mothers, child and adolescent psychiatric patients, children affected by post-traumatic stress disorder, bulimic girls, sufferers of fibromyalgia, burn patients, and the elderly.[24] A TRI study is in progress that examines the effect of full-body relaxation massages on women who have completed treatment for breast cancer. It seems safe to assume that similar results will be attained with this group.

The effect of massage on the fatigue that accompanies cancer is one of the least studied issues. Patients who receive massage at Oregon Health Sciences University are asked to rate fatigue on a 1–5 Likert Scale before and after each massage. The data from ninety-three patients found that 73 percent perceived a decrease in their fatigue following the massage. The group average prior to massage was a 3. Following the session the group average dropped to a 2 (5 = severe, 1 = mild).

Massage therapy can play a significant role in reunifying the whole person with themselves, and with the human community.

— ANNETTE CHAMNESS, C.M.T.

Wilkinson's study is the only one that specifically asked patients about quality of life.[9] Nearly all of the recipients in that investigation reported the four weekly massages did improve this aspect of their life. Quality of living is a complex issue composed of many interrelated factors. Cancer pain is the most studied topic with regard to massage, but how this translates to activity rates or coping strategies is unknown. The effect of bodywork on cancer depression and fatigue has yet to be addressed. Instinct suggests that these factors will be positively affected by skilled touch. Common sense and anecdotal evidence also hint that massage, combined with standard care and other adjuvant therapies, will help patients better perform daily functions, remain active, have a more positive self-image, increase their energy, and have a higher quality of life. In the end, this might also translate to increased survival.

PSYCHOSOCIAL SUPPORT

Evidence shows that psychosocial factors can also influence the quality of life of some cancer patients.[23] Interventions such as group support have been shown to improve patients' emotional well-being. Dr. David Spiegel, a Stanford psychiatrist, was surprised to find it even affected length of survival. In his study of 86 women with metastatic breast cancer, Spiegel found that the group who attended a weekly support group for a one year period, in addition to receiving routine oncological care, lived twice as long as the group who only received standard medical care.[25]

Fawzy et al. also found psychiatric intervention given early after surgery extended the survival rate in malignant melanoma patients.[26] The experimental group participated in a six week program that included education, stress management, coping skills, and psychological support. Five to six years later, this group showed less reoccurrence (7 out of 34 patients) and fewer deaths (3 out of 34). For control patients the numbers were 13 out of 34 and 10 out of 34, respectively.

Spiegel hypothesized that group involvement may assist patients to comply more strictly with their medical treatment, or it may reduce depression, resulting in improved appetite and diet. Patients in his group also learned to use hypnosis for pain management, which may have helped them to remain more active. Group involvement also provides a forum for patients to voice their feelings. Justice reports that in a study of women with metastatic breast cancer, those who were expressive of negative feelings and showed their unhappiness remained alive after a year more often than women who kept their feelings to themselves. Having a place to share one's feelings may also relieve anxiety and depression in some individuals. Because there is a strong relationship between pain and the emotions of depression, anxiety, and anger,[3,6,12] relief of these feelings through group support may also reduce pain.[4]

For most of us, sickness is to varying extents a plunge into radical aloneness. We try to communicate to those who are closest to us, hoping they can share our burden, but our suffering remains maddeningly private.

— MARC IAN BARASCH,
THE HEALING PATH

Scientists are beginning to speculate that a connection also exists between the immune system and expressing emotions. In "Immune Power Personality," Henry Dreher refers to two studies that indicate cancer spreads more rapidly in breast cancer patients who repress their emotions or have a sense of helplessness. Patients who are able to express their feelings and needs, and obtain support from family and friends, live longer or have higher rates of remission than those who deny their emotions.[27] It is therefore logical to theorize that any intervention that creates a supportive atmosphere conducive to the sharing of feelings will be helpful in boosting the immune system and therefore have a positive effect on the disease.

Support groups give many patients a place to share their emotions, but others are unable to open up in this atmosphere. For these patients, the private, nurturing environment of a massage session might provide the environment necessary for them to share the emotions that accompany such a devastating situation. The women in Menard's investigation rated the massage sessions high in terms of emotional support, as did those in Wilkinson's study. Half of the patients in the Wilkinson investigation reported the primary benefit of the massages had been emotional, and that being able to talk about their fears and worries to someone who understood was a great help. In an ideal world, people with cancer would have equal access to support groups and touch therapy. Perhaps the two used in combination would yield an even greater benefit.

A SUMMARY OF RESEARCH

The fact that massage research is being conducted with people who have cancer is, in and of itself, an important event. Health care institutions such as the University of Miami Medical School's Touch Research Institute and Marie Curie Cancer Centre in England, or agencies that award grants such as the American Massage Therapy Association and the National Institute of Health's Office of Alternative Medicine, would never approve research that has the potential to harm patients; nor would researchers seek permission to engage in such study. While some of the studies are lacking in terms of sample size, methodology, and statistical analysis, the oncology expertise of each of the investigators must be acknowledged. All of the researchers possess impeccable credentials, from that of radiation oncologist, to professors of psychiatry at the Dartmouth Medical School Center for Psycho-Oncology Research, to British and American oncology nurses, and nursing school professors, to name just some. The bodywork community must fashion its clinical practice around the knowledge of these experts.

Normally, research is reported in reviews of literature in a cursory way. Offering the results in greater detail, as well as information about the subjects and methodology, is instructive to the reader and creates a more detailed picture in the mind's eye. And because some practitioners are tentative about working with this population, greater detail should provide additional reassurance that most of the medical community now views massage as an acceptable part of cancer patients' treatment regimen. Hopefully too, it will get the research juices flowing in an increased number of bodyworkers. Until now, touch therapists have not conducted and seldom even participated in research with cancer patients. Largely, the studies have been conducted by nurses, psychologists, physicians, and other medical staff. Bodyworkers have much to contribute to research, as they have an approach that is unique from that of other health care providers.

Existing Research

The majority of research with cancer patients has been conducted in the area of Swedish Massage and Manual Lymphatic Drainage, with one study one examining Myofascial Release. The effect of Therapeutic Touch has been examined with hospitalized patients, and as an analgesic, but not with cancer patients specifically. Most of the studies look at the use of these techniques as comfort measures or quality of life issues.

Swedish Massage

...science is confirming what we know in our hearts: that, as psychiatrist James Gordon put it, "massage is medicine."

— George Howe Colt

Denise Tope, Assistant Professor of Psychiatry at Dartmouth Medical School, researched the effect of two or more massages on 104 patients over a four year period.[7] The subjects were of two types, either general cancer patients (40 percent) or autologous bone marrow transplant (ABMT) patients (60 percent). (In ABMT the patient donates her own bone marrow prior to undergoing high doses of chemotherapy.) The massages were administered by a Licensed Practical Nurse, were limited to 30 minutes, and commonly included work on the back, shoulders, neck and feet. Upon discharge, patients completed a self-report questionnaire. "Relaxation" or "release of muscle tension" were mentioned by 99 percent of the patients. In addition, 35 percent commented on improved mood or sense of well-being, 22 percent mentioned assistance symptom management (control of pain, inflammation, nausea) and 15 percent felt a decreased sense of isolation. None of the patients made reference to any negative effects of massage.

Tope et al. focused on ABMT patients because of the severity of treatment-related symptoms. "ABMT patients generally experience side effects from toxicity and immunosuppression associated with the procedure, such as high fevers, nausea and vomiting, painful skin rashes, and debilitating fatigue, along with other idiosyncratic symptoms." In addition, they remain in the hospital for extended periods of time (at least three weeks), and for a portion of that time are unable to leave the protected environment. These factors, along with the ever-present potential of mortality can increase anxiety and depression in these patients. More data will be forthcoming on the topic of massage therapy for post-bone marrow transplant distress, as this researcher received an NIH grant in 1993 to further her exploration into this area.

Sally Sims, a British nurse, researched the use of slow stroke back massage on six female patients receiving radiation therapy for breast cancer.[28] Pre- and post-measures were taken with the subjects serving as their own controls. Thirteen symptoms were measured on a 1–5 scale: nausea (frequency and intensity), pain (frequency and intensity), appetite, insomnia, fatigue, bowel pattern, concentration, appearance, breathing, outlook and cough. Each massage lasted ten minutes and consisted of slow, gentle, rhythmical strokes using both hands over the back. One group of three patients received massage for three consecutive days. The following week they were scheduled for a 10 minute rest for three consecutive days. Group 2 received the massage and the control intervention (10 minute rest) in reverse order. Three of the six subjects reported an improvement in total symptom distress following the 10 minute rest. Five out of six reported a greater improvement in total symptom distress following the massage. Sims analyzed the data from several different angles. However, for the most part the differences between the massage and the 10 minute rest were not statistically significant. The researcher suggested that the small sample size and large number of symptom variables may have contributed to the results. She also comments that individual patient needs were not taken into account, and "the giving of massage within a research setting may have undermined its true effects."

Andrea Ferrell-Tory and Orpha Glick, faculty members of the University of Iowa College of Nursing, examined the effects of massage on pain perception, anxiety, and relaxation in nine male patients experiencing significant cancer pain.[8] The subjects had a wide variety of cancers, esophageal, rectal, prostate, stomach, and lung, as well as leukemia and mixed nodular lymphoma. Five of the patients had also been diagnosed with metastases to distant sites. Thirty minute massages were given on two consecutive evenings. Massage consisted of effleurage and petrissage to the feet, back, neck, and shoulders, plus myofascial trigger points (localized tender spots) located in the upper, middle, and lower trapezius. "Once TPs [trigger points] were located, slow, milking strokes of increasing pressure were utilized along the length of the effected muscle to gradually reduce the pain associated with the TP." Immediately before and after the massage subjects completed self-reports with regard to pain and relaxation. In addition, heart rate (HR), respiratory rate (R), and blood pressure (BP) were taken just before, immediately after, and 10 minutes after massage. Subjects' level of pain perception was reduced by an average of 60 percent, anxiety by 24 percent, and feelings of relaxation increased by 58 percent. HR, R, and BP "tended to decrease from baseline, providing further indication of relaxation."

Sally Weinrich and Martin Weinrich, from the College of Nursing and the Department of Epidemiology and Biostatistics at the University of South Carolina, researched the effect of massage on cancer pain.[10] Twenty-eight hospitalized patients (18 men and 10 women) were assigned to a massage or control group. The massage group was given a 10 minute Swedish back massage from senior nursing students, while the control group received a 10 minute visit by the same students. The control was intended to account for the possibility that any effect might be due to the attention the patients were receiving. Immediately before and after the intervention patients rated their pain on a Visual Analogue Scale, the two end points being "no pain" and "pain as bad as it could possibly be." There was no significant difference in pain for males or females in the control group. For males in the massage group there was a significant decrease in pain immediately after the massage. However, for females there was not. The authors note that the men had a high level of self-reported pain prior to the massage, while the women initially had a low level. This led them to wonder if there are differences in how each gender copes with and perceives pain, or if massage has greater social acceptability among one gender more than the other.

Nurse researcher, Susie Wilkinson, of the Marie Curie Cancer Centre in Liverpool, England, studied the effects of a series of four weekly, full-body massages on the quality of life for patients with advanced cancer.[9] The most common sites of cancer in the participants were breast, lung, gynecological, and head and neck. Fifty-six out of the 87 subjects had metastatic disease. Patients were referred to the project primarily for anxiety and tension, followed by pain and depression.

Sixty-eight percent of the massage recipients returned their questionnaires. All of them said that relaxation was a positive result of massage. Aside from relaxation, 33 percent reported pain reduction, while 20 percent reported other physical benefits such as decreased edema, increased mobility, and improved skin condition. About half indicated that the positive aspects of the massages had been mainly physical, while the other half reported the primary benefit to be emotional or spiritual. One of the important emotional themes that surfaced for patients was the benefit of being given time and attention specifically for them. For some, the massage sessions were a time out from the illness. For others the massages helped them to cope better with their situation.

It was an important aspect of the massages that patients were able to talk about their cancer experiences during the sessions. One patient said that, "The feeling of warmth and caring at the center is very beneficial to me. Talking of my fears and worries... to someone

The act of massage unites heaven and earth, spirit and matter, divine and mundane.

— G.M.

who understands is a great help to me. I feel I have benefited from the fact that I am not alone with cancer anymore."

Only eight patients indicated that there had been something they didn't like about the massages. These included the smell of the oil, or having oil on their hair and faces, or the initial embarrassment. Eight patients felt they had acquired some self-help skills and information. This gave them a feeling of control over events which enabled them to cope more effectively with their illness.

As part of the same study, Wilkinson examined the differences between massage performed with aromatherapy oil and without it. Aromatherapy is the use of fragrances to enhance well-being. In this case the essential oil Roman Chamomile was added to the unscented almond oil used on one of the groups, while the other group received massage with almond oil only. Roman Chamomile was chosen because of its abilities to act as an analgesic, as an anti-inflammatory, as an antiseptic, as an antispasmodic, as a diuretic, as a digestive, and for its ability to relieve gas from the intestinal tract. The massage technique, performed by three nurses with specialized training, was the same for both groups.[29,30]

Patients were surveyed on quality of life measures such as physical status (lack of energy, sore muscles, pain, etc.), psychological distress, ability to perform daily activities, and overall quality of life. Both groups showed a statistically significant decrease in anxiety. The scores of the aromatherapy group reached statistical significance on several of the measurement inventories: global quality of life, physical symptoms, and psychological distress. The group that received only massage showed a deterioration in the physical status measurements and improvement in psychological and quality of life scores. The scores did not, however, reach statistical significance. Both groups had a deterioration in the activities subscale score.[30] Dr. Wilkinson and her colleagues will begin a new study in March of 1998 at four cancer centers in England. This investigation, a randomized controlled trial, will look at the efficacy of aromatherapy massage and relaxation therapy in patients' quality of life.

Martha Brown Menard investigated the effect of massage on 15 women who had undergone a hysterectomy because of probable malignant disease.[11] The 15 women in the experimental group received standard care plus a daily massage. Fifteen other women received only standard post-surgical care. Subjects in the massage group received 45 minute massage sessions beginning the first day after surgery and continuing throughout hospitalization. Patients initially received massage to the head, neck, shoulders, feet, legs, hands, and arms using primarily effleurage and petrissage. Once they were comfortable in a side-lying position, the back was included. Therapists also incorporated acupressure to points along the bladder meridian.

Menard hypothesized that massage would promote faster recovery from surgery. Although statistical significance was not quite reached for many of the variables examined, the trend, when compared with the standard care group, was toward a faster and better recovery. Patients' cortisol levels, systolic blood pressure (the top number), and pain ratings were all lower; they had less anxiety and depression and used less pain medication; bowel function and sleep were better; and the length of stay was shorter by half a day. One variable that did reach statistical significance was the use of additional medical services during the four week follow-up period. Five of the patients in the control group required visits to their physician for surgically related problems. Meanwhile, no one in the massage group needed an additional visit to the doctor. This last finding, as well as the decreased use of pain medication during hospitalization, is financially significant.

Pauline King, a mental health nurse at The James Cancer Hospital and Research Institute in Columbus, Ohio, researched the effect of massage on pain and anxiety of hospitalized cancer patients in conjunction with the use of prescribed pain medication. Subjects in the experimental group received one 15 minute massage approximately two hours after the administration of pain medication. Effleurage and petrissage was given to the hands, feet, head, and neck. The control group underwent the same protocol, except someone sat with them for 15 minutes instead of giving massage.[31] King found that a 15 minute massage given after pain medication provided no statistically significant relief from pain. Because patients' pain at The James Cancer Hospital was so well managed by pharmacological means, the investigator felt there was little room for improvement. The analysis, however, did point toward a reduction in anxiety that nearly reached statistical significance.[32]

MYOFASCIAL RELEASE

Following a lumpectomy and radiation, most breast cancer patients have an excellent outcome. However, a few patients have chest wall tenderness due to fibrosis which is not responsive to anti-inflammatory medication. Radiation oncologist Dr.John Crawford studied twelve such women to see if the Myofascial Release (MFR) technique would be effective in relieving this type of chronic pain.[33]

The fascia is a tough connective tissue that spreads without interruption through out the body from head to foot. Trauma, such as surgery or inflammation can cause the fascia to scar or harden, which can cause pressure on nerves, muscles, blood vessels, bones, or organs, creating pain and decreased range of motion. Because fascia extends throughout the entire body, injury to it in one area can put tension on adjacent or even distant areas. MFR practitioners describe their technique as a gentle application of sustained pressure to the fascial restrictions.

The MFR treatments in this study were given by Physical or Occupational Therapists three times a week for three weeks. The sessions were begun two months after the patients finished their medical treatment to insure that no active cancer remained. This was determined from CT scans. All 12 participants experience some pain relief. Eight of the 12 had complete or near complete relief, while the other four reported an improvement. Patients were followed up for 4-65 months. Two people required retreatment with MFR, resulting in relief of their symptoms.

Hopefully this modality will be studied further. MFR may have use for all breast cancer patients whose cancer is inactive, not just as a last resort but as a front line treatment. Perhaps integrating it into the rehabilitation program of more breast cancer patients would allow them to take lower doses of pain medication. Drugs not only have significant side effects but are also expensive.

LYMPHATIC DRAINAGE THERAPIES

One of the side effects of cancer or its treatment can be lymphedema. In fact, cancer is the most common cause of lymphedema in the U.S., with breast cancer, melanomas, and lymphomas most frequently associated.[34] Lymphedema, the excess accumulation of fluid and protein in the tissues, may be caused when lymphatic vessels become blocked by scar tissue following radiation treatment or by tumors; become damaged from chemotherapy; or become swollen when the normal flow of lymphatic fluid cannot be accommodated after the removal of lymph nodes. According to Manual Lymphatic Drainage (MLD) instructor, Robert Harris, "When proteins are not removed from the connective tissue by the lymph system, they tend to become organized and fibrotic, making removal much more difficult. Also, proteins exert a colloid osmotic pressure, attracting water [through cell membranes] into the connective tissue and causing edema. The longer the proteins sit there, the more difficult the problem becomes, so it is important to begin treatment as soon as possible to clean out the accumulated proteins".[35]

A variety of lymphatic drainage therapies exist. These interventions have been shown to relieve edema, fibrosis (the process of adhesion or scar tissue formation), and the accompanying pain and discomfort. Dr. Vodder's Manual Lymphatic Drainage technique is probably the best known in the U.S., however, all of the variations of this genre are effective. These techniques, which are regarded as routine treatment in European hospitals, are considered to be a specialized form of massage that use a gentle, rhythmic, pumping movement as in MLD,[36] or a "steady, gentle, wave-like motion" as with Dr. Chikly's Lymphatic Drainage Therapy.[31] Lymphatic massage alone is not enough to resolve lymphedema – bandaging, compressive garments, exercises, and skin care must be

Giving massage to another is a form of communication in which the hands do much of the talking.

— TEDI DUNN
AND MARIAN WILLIAMS,
MASSAGE THERAPY GUIDELINES
FOR HOSPITAL AND HOME CARE

used in conjunction with it. Dr. Vodder calls this part of his treatment regimen, Combined Decongestive Therapy (CDT). Medicare refers to the entire process, including the massage component, as Complex Decongestive Therapy (CDP).

Many physicians prescribe the use of a pneumatic compression machine for their lymphedema patients. The literature presents evidence that these devices produce good results in early Grade 1 lymphedema. P. O. Hutzchenreuter, an Austrian doctor, and Hildegard Wittlinger cite a study in which patients showed a 30 percent decrease in volume after two months of daily treatment with a pneumatic device, while they were able to achieve a 20 percent reduction in 62 post-mastectomy patients using MLD and CDT daily for three weeks.[38]

Australian physician Ian Bunce and others evaluated a multi-modal approach that included a manual lymphatic drainage technique, pneumatic compression, bandaging, and education about the post-mastectomy condition.[39] The participants were 25 women who had confirmed or suspected loco-regional cancer, with no evidence of metastasis. There was an average interval of six years since surgery. Patients were excluded whose lymphedema or illness was so severe that independently managing their condition was unlikely.

Treatments were given three hours a day, five days a week, for four weeks. Each patient and a companion were taught how to perform massage and bandage the effected limb. Excess limb volume decreased about 40 percent immediately after the treatment and by over 50 percent at the six month follow-up. This achievement remained stable at the 12 month follow-up. The modalities that required assistance, massage and bandaging, decreased more following the treatment series than did exercise or compression sleeve wearing. This multi-modal, self-managed form of rehabilitation would seem to be one way of receiving the benefits of therapy while containing the cost to patients and the community.

Zanolla et al., from the Department of Pain Therapy and Rehabilitation in Milan, Italy, investigated the efficacy of three different methods of treating lymphedema following a mastectomy.[40] Three groups of 20 women were given one of three methods of treatment: pneumatic compression with a uniform pressure, pneumatic compression with differentiated pressures, and Manual Lymphatic Drainage. The pneumatic massage was used six hours a day for one week. The MLD group received massage for one hour, three times a week for a month. Each group also wore a compression sleeve during the day. Three months following the end of treatment, a statistically significant, permanent improvement was achieved for those receiving uniform pneumatic massage and Manual Lymphatic Drainage massage. The group receiving differentiated pressure had very little reduction in edema.

At one time compression pumps were thought to be the most effective way to remove excess fluid and protein build-up from tissues. This traditional approach is now in question. While pumps are helpful for Grade 1 lymphedema, they are of little use for longer-lasting conditions or where the tissue has become fibrotic. In addition they can cause unwanted side effects. Lymphedema may pool in areas that were previously normal, such as in the trunk, genitals, or the opposite limb.[41]

Compression sleeves have been found to be an effective component in management of lymphedema. However, women sometimes find them to be uncomfortable, so are reluctant to wear them. In her study at the Wessex Cancer Centre in England, Rachel Hornsby examined whether wearing a compression sleeve was an essential part of treatment for lymphedema, or whether exercise, skin care, self-massage, and education were sufficient.[42] Twenty-five women were randomly placed in either an experimental (14) or control group (11). Both groups received instruction in self-massage, an exercise regimen, skin care, and education about lymphedema. In addition, those in the experimental group were fitted with elastic compression sleeves which they were asked to wear day and night.

During the first four week interval, 12 of the 14 experimental participants had a reduction in swelling; the other two showed an increase. Only four of the 11 control subjects had reduced swelling, with three having an increase. All of the patients reported that even when there was no fluid loss, their arm felt less heavy and more mobile from doing the exercises and massage. Perhaps these patients had not been moving their arms, causing stiffness from a lack of activity. Hornsby's study suggests that wearing a compression sleeve may be a necessary component along with exercise and massage in the self-management of lymphedema. Further research is needed to compare the effectiveness of self-management of lymphedema versus treatment by health care professionals who can administer more skillful modalities such as lymph drainage techniques.

Lymphedema often occurs much later following surgery. The women in Hutzschenreuter's study had their surgeries 1–26 years prior to being referred for MLD, with the average being 3.5 years. Robert Harris reported the case history of a woman whose mastectomy had been nine years prior to consulting him. The lymphedema had begun two years following surgery when swollen axillary nodes were removed. The patient was eager to receive MLD rather than be "hooked up to a milking machine at a place where she would be reminded every time that she had cancer." When she began treatment the right arm was 40 percent larger than the left. Following ten treatments over a one month period, it was only 16 percent larger. For this patient, like many others, treatments must be on-going because of the lymph node removal. The frequency of sessions can be greatly reduced though, once the majority of fluid has been removed.

Just as the massage therapists's hands contour to the physical shape of the physical body, so do the Attunement practitioner's hands conform themselves to the natural subtle energy profile of the etheric body.

— JACLYN STEIN HENDERSON,
THE HEALING POWER OF
ATTUNEMENT THERAPY:
STORIES AND PRACTICE

Dr. Michael Brennan presented a case history of new onset lymphedema which occurred 39 years after a radical mastectomy.[34] The swelling was believed to have been brought on by infection due to daily finger sticks to test blood sugar. The patient's lymphedema was completely reduced after one month of wearing compression garments and administering massage to herself.

More and more, manual lymphatic massage is becoming the primary intervention for removing excess lymph with compression pumps used as an adjunct. Manual methods are advantagous not only in their ability to lower limb swelling, they also re-train the body to open collateral lymphatic channels, and can direct the lymphatic fluid toward adjacent functioning areas.[41] Additionally, they can also improve scar consistency, stimulate revascularization, promote mobility, and increase skin elasticity.[38,43] And not to be minimized is the human contact and caring touch that hands-on treatment provides, The sense of being cared for after a traumatic and often disfiguring surgery is immensely healing.

THERAPEUTIC TOUCH

Therapeutic Touch (T.T.) is often referred to as a form of energy healing or a subtle energy technique. It works with the energy field of the body, sometimes known as the aura, rather than with muscle and connective tissue or with the physiological processes of the body. When practicing this modality, the therapist often does not touch the physical body, but directs energy with the hands positioned a few inches above the body. Patricia Heidt distinguishes T.T. from casual touch in that T.T. is touch given with the intent to help or heal patients.[44]

Some study has been made by nurses from various nursing school faculty of Therapeutic Touch's effect on hospitalized patients and people in pain. Despite the fact that none of these projects examined cancer patients specifically, the results of these studies would seem to be applicable to hospitalized cancer patients or those effected by cancer pain. Unfortunately, the data regarding T.T. is mixed and is still somewhat controversial. Therapeutic Touch has not yet provided sufficient evidence that it is any more effective than a placebo.[45]

The studies cited by Arlen Jurgens and others are a perfect example of the inconclusiveness within Therapeutic Touch research. Parks evaluated the effect of T.T. on the anxiety of elderly hospitalized patients and also found no significant difference compared to a mimic treatment. On the other hand, Heidt reported a significant decrease in the anxiety of hospitalized cardiovascular patients who received Therapeutic Touch compared to those who received either casual touch or verbal interaction. When Janet Quinn replicated Heidt's research she did not find a significant decrease in the anxiety of those patients.[45]

Therese Meehan reports on a study by Hale regarding Therapeutic Touch with hospitalized adults.[46] Like Parks, no significant decrease was found in the anxiety of these people. In her own research, Meehan looked at the effect of T.T. on patients who were experiencing pain following major abdominal surgery. One hundred-eight subjects were randomly assigned to a Therapeutic Touch group, a placebo control intervention that mimicked T.T., or the standard narcotic intervention. The Therapeutic Touch group received a standardized five minute procedure from nurses who were experienced T.T. practitioners. The placebo intervention was also five minutes long, but the nurse only mimicked the hand movements of T.T., and made no attempt to assume a meditative state of awareness, had no intention to assist or attune to the subject, or to consciously direct the flow of energy as is done in a Therapeutic Touch session. Pain measurements were taken just prior to the intervention and one hour following.

Meehan hypothesized that Therapeutic Touch would significantly decrease postoperative pain compared to the placebo intervention. However, this was not the case. The T.T. group did show decreased pain compared to the mimic group, but it did not quite reach statistical significance. Secondary analyses suggest that T.T. may decrease the amount of pain medication needed compared to the placebo group. As would be expected, standard pain medication had the greatest effect. Meehan suggests that Therapeutic Touch administered in conjunction with narcotics may potentiate their effect. Possibly a longer session than the five-minute intervention used in this project and other T.T. studies would produce the desired results. The nurses commented that with most subjects the time period was too short, that they were just getting going when it was time to stop.

Research by Nancy Kramer of hospitalized children, ages two weeks to two years, showed T.T. to significantly decrease stress compared to casual touching.[47] Her study measured pulse, galvanic skin response, and peripheral skin temperature when the children were observed to be in stress, and again three and six minutes after the intervention was begun. Therapeutic Touch proved to be effective in reducing the time needed to calm children after a stressful experience such as a procedure.

Anecdotal reports suggest that T.T. applied before and after surgery decreases surgically induced anemia and fatigue and speeds up wound healing.[4] Nurses who use Therapeutic Touch believe that it increases relaxation and relieves pain and anxiety. "It is difficult not to believe in these effects when they are so frequently reported by patients. Patients treated for pain, often only partially relieved by narcotics, frequently report that although they still have pain after treatment, it no longer bothers them."[45] Wright suggests that T.T. is effective for cancer patients, especially those with bone metastases, who cannot tolerate actual physical touch. It can reduce the sense of isolation and create comfort and relaxation in the patient.[4] Bodywork practitioners intuitively know these reports to be true, but as of yet, no research has been reported in the formal literature to support the claims.

In the book, *A Doctor's Guide to Therapeutic Touch*, Dr. Susan Wager relates her experience of patients recovering more rapidly from surgery when treated with T.T. beforehand.[48] They come out of anaesthesia more quickly and incisions heal faster. Those on a chemotherapy and/or radiation regimen benefit by incurring less nausea, vomiting, and diarrhea, and increased energy. Dr. Wager makes the following suggestions about the use of Therapeutic Touch with cancer patients:

1. Administer T.T. before chemotherapy and radiation. This has been shown to reduce the side effects.

2. Give sessions on a regular basis to increase energy and relieve symptoms as they occur.

3. Direct energy over the solar plexus area to help alleviate nausea and anxiety.

4. Also direct energy over the liver and lymph nodes, as they are often areas to which cancer will metastasize.

5. Approach the patient as being whole, rather than focusing on the organ or region where the tumor is located.

REIKI

Another subtle energy technique often used with cancer patients is Reiki. Like Therapeutic Touch, it too is referred to as a modern-day laying on of hands. Unlike T.T., which believes that energy is transferred from the practitioner to the recipient and that the flow of energy can be directed, Reiki operates under the philosophy that the practitioner is merely a conduit for universal life energy. During a Reiki session the practitioner's hands most often are in direct contact with the recipient's body, rather than being held above as in a T.T. session.

Very little research exists with regard to this discipline. Wendy Wetzel, using first degree Reiki practitioners, replicated Dolores Krieger's 1975 study on the effect of Therapeutic touch on hemoglobin levels.[49] Her findings indicated significant improvement in hemoglobin levels of a group of 48 Reiki trainees 24 hours after their training compared with the levels of a control group of 10 medical professionals who did not receive the training.

Libby Barnett and Maggie Chambers offer anecdotal accounts in their book, *Reiki Energy Medicine*, of Reiki being administered to a teacher prior to her bone marrow transplant, to 54 year-old woman with a brain tumor as part of preparation for surgery, and a 67 year-old man who was extremely agitated during the postoperative phase following a craniotomy for a tumor.[50] They report that nurses often tell them stories of using Reiki when standard procedures have not worked. "Surgeons and nurse anesthetists find Reiki to be helpful pre-, intra-, and postoperatively. The Reiki touch helps the anesthetist to connect quickly with patient while simultaneously reducing the patient's anxiety regarding the impending procedure. The anesthetist's job is much easier when the patient is less fearful." Patient's receiving chemotherapy have commented on feeling less distress and discomfort when Reiki is part of their care plan.

The loving touch, like music, often utters the things that cannot be spoken.
— ASHLEY MONTAGU

Subtle energy techniques such as Reiki are advantageous in that they are simple, easy to learn, and can be self-administered more easily compared to other bodywork modalities. In her book, *The 'Reiki' Factor in the Radiance Technique*, Barbara Ray devotes an entire chapter to the effects The Radiance Technique (TRT) has had on cancer patients who took the TRT training and later used it on themselves.[51] Besides feeling more energy, hope, and tranquility, patients were able to reduce their dependence on analgesics, gained weight, prolonged their lives, ameliorated the side effects of chemotherapy, accelerated the healing process following surgery, and required shorter hospital stays.

SHEN

SHEN, an acronym for Specific Human Energy Nexus, is a lesser known form of energy work, which, like Reiki, uses a pressureless, non-invasive touch. *The Handbook of Shen* cites its use with several cancer patients whose white blood count had dropped to low levels. Following the session, the white blood counts had risen.[52]

RESEARCH IN PROGRESS

Several research projects are in progress as *Medicine Hands* goes to the printer. Densie Tope received a grant in 1993 from the Office of Alternative Medicine to research the effects of massage on bone marrow transplant patients. Energy therapist Julie Motz has received a grant to perform subtle energy therapy before, during, and after breast cancer surgery for 15 women.[53] The Touch Research Institute has two studies underway.[24] In one investigation parents are being taught to massage their children who have cancer. The second study is examining the effect of full-body relaxation massages on women who have finished treatment for stage one or stage two breast cancers. The focus is on immune measures and psychological response. Tiffany Field, director of the Touch Research Institute, reported that because women with breast cancer have shown such a "whopping increase" in natural killer and other immune cells as a result of receiving massage, she wants to do studies with all kinds of cancer patients.[54]

IDEAS FOR FUTURE RESEARCH

1. Examine the relationship between massage and remaining active.

2. Examine the effect of combining massage with standard pain interventions.

3. Compare the number of doctor's office visits, the amount of money spent on pain medications, and frequency of re-hospitalization on an experimental group that receives bi-monthly massage and a control group that receives only standard medical care.

4. Compare the effects between differing touch modalities.

5. Modify David Spiegel's study so that massage is substituted for the weekly support group.

6. Examine the difference in efficacy between sessions of different lengths, such as 15 minutes versus 45 minutes.

7. Compare sessions given by nursing staff with those given by professional touch practitioners.

8. Examine the effect of daily massage on the length of hospital stay of bone marrow transplant patients.

9. Examine the effect of regular bodywork sessions on patients' perception of fatigue.

10. Examine the effect massage would have on the self-image of chemotherapy or breast cancer patients.

11. Examine the effect of cumulative massages.

12. Examine the effect of individually tailored sessions compared to standardized ones.

FINAL THOUGHTS

We instinctively know that intentional, loving touch is good medicine. Most certainly the study of bodywork will continue to prove its benefit for cancer patients. This may not be enough however. Many Western cultures value prosperity first, with compassion and quality of life as runners-up. Those who hold the purse strings want proof that massage has monetary advantages before fully integrating it into mainstream health care. They need to see hard numbers showing that it decreases hospital stays, reduces the need for medication, or allows people to return to work sooner. It is not enough to show that massage can create hope, can ameliorate the symptoms of disease and its treatment, or calm the body and soul.

Putting the responsibility for this situation onto mainstream medicine or insurance companies would be easy, but they are only a reflection of ourselves...our beliefs and practices. Perhaps it isn't the insurance companies that need persuading, maybe it's all of us, patients, family members, and practitioners that need to be convinced massage is worthwhile, whether it shortens hospital stays or not. Why isn't it enough to ease the burden on family caregivers, to provide relief from the nausea caused by chemotherapy, or to assuage the loneliness of five weeks in a bone marrow transplant unit? Aren't we worth it? Massage is not a luxury but a necessary part of a complete healing regimen and should be included in "standard care."

ACKNOWLEDGMENT

Parts of this chapter were adapted from "Massage for Cancer Patients: A Review of Nursing Research," *Massage Therapy Journal*®, Vol. 34, No.3, Summer 1995. Reprinted with permission of the American Massage Therapy Association®.

REFERENCES

1. Foley, K. Controlling the Pain of Cancer. *Scientific American.* 1996; 275(3):164-165.

2. Daut, R.L. and C.S. Cleeland. The Prevalence and Severity of Pain in Cancer. *Cancer.* 1982;50(9):1913-1918.

3. Arathuzik, D. The Appraisal of Pain and Coping in Cancer Patients. *Western Journal of Nursing Research.* 1991; 13(6): 714-731.

4. Wright, S. The Use of Therapeutic Touch in the Management of Pain. *Nursing Clinics of North America.* 1987; 22(3):705-714.

5. Physician Role Model Program Encourages an Aggressive Approach to Managing Cancer Pain. *Trends (Medical College of Wisconsin).* Autumn 1991. p.14.

6.   Dorrepaal, K.L.; N.K. Aaronson; and F. Van Dam. Pain
Experience and Pain Management Among Hospitalized Cancer
Patients. *Cancer*. 1989;63(3):593-598.

7.   Tope, D.M.; D.M. Hann; and B. Pinkson. Massage therapy: An
old intervention comes of age. *Quality of Life – A Nursing Challenge*.
1994;3:14-18.

8.   Ferrell-Torry, A.T. and O.J. Glick. The use of therapeutic
massage as a nursing intervention to modify anxiety and the
perception of cancer pain. *Cancer Nursing*. 1993;16:93-101.

9.   Wilkinson, S. Get The Massage. *Nursing Times*. 1996;92(34):61-
64.

10. Weinrich, S.P. and M.C. Weinrich. The effect of massage on
pain in cancer patients. *Applied Nursing Research*. 1990;3(4):140-
145.

11. Menard, M. The Effect of Therapeutic Massage on Post-Surgical
Outcomes. Doctoral dissertation, University of Virginia. 1995

12. Twycross, R. and S. Fairfield. Pain in Far-advanced Cancer. *Pain*.
1982;14:303-310.

13. Rhiner, M.; B.R. Ferrell; B.A. Ferrell; and M.M. Grant. A
structured nondrug intervention program for cancer pain. *Cancer
Practice*. 1993;1(2):137-143.

14. Ferrell, B.R. and C. Schneider. Experience and Management of
Cancer Pain at Home. *Cancer Nursing*. 1988; 11(2): 84-90.

15. Ahles, T.A.; E.B. Blanchard; and J.C. Ruckdeschel. The
Multidimensional Nature of Cancer-Related Pain. *Pain*.
1983;17:277-288.

16. Dalton, J.; T. Toomey; and M. Workman. Pain Relief for Cancer
Patients. *Cancer Nursing*. 1988; 11(6): 322-328.

17. Scott, D.; D. Donahue; R. Mastrovito; and T. Hakes. The
Antiemetic Effect of Clinical Relaxation: Report of an Exploratory
Pilot Study. *Journal of Psychosocial Oncology*. 1983; 1(1):71-83.

18. Ferrell, B.; M. Cohen; M. Rhiner; and A. Rozek. Pain as a
Metaphor for Illness Part II: Family Caregivers' Management of
Pain. *Oncology Nursing Forum*. 1991;18(8):1315-1321.

19. Degner, L. and D. Barkwell. Nonanalgesic Approaches to Pain
Control. *Cancer Nursing*. 1991;14(2):105-111.

20. Barbour, L.; D. Maguire; and K. Kirchhoff. Nonanalgesic
Methods of Pain Control Used by Cancer Outpatients. *Oncology
Nursing Forum*. 1986;13(6):56-60.

21. MacVicar, M. and M. Winningham. Promoting the Functional
Capacity of Cancer Patients. *The Cancer Bulletin*. 1986;38(5):235-
238.

22. Weiner, E. Quality-of-Life Research in Patients with Breast Cancer. *Cancer Supplement*. 1994;74(1):410-415.

23. Justice, B. Evidence of Psychosocial Influence in Disease Onset and Outcome. *The Cancer Bulletin*. 1986;38(5):241.

24. Touch Research Institute Studies. *Hospital-Based Massage Newsletter*. 1997;3(1):15-19.

25. Spiegel, D. Effect of Psychosocial Treatment on Survival of Patients with Metastatic Breast Cancer. *The Lancet*. October 14, 1989. P. 888-891.

26. Fawzy, I,; N.W. Fawzy; C.S. Hyun; R. Elashoff; D. Guthrie; J.L. Fahey; and D.L. Morton. Malignant Melanoma: Effects of an Early Structured Psychiatric Intervention, Coping, and Affective State on Recurrence and Survival 6 Years Later. *Archives of General Psychiatry*. 1993;50:681-689.

27. Dreher, H. Immune Power Personality. *Noetic Sciences Review*. Autumn 1996. p.12-16.

28. Sims, S. Slow stroke back massage for cancer patients. *Nursing Times*. 1986;82(13):47-50.

29. Wilkinson, S. Aromatherapy and Massage in Palliative Care. *International Journal of Palliative Nursing*. 1995;1(1):21-30.

30. Wilkinson, S. An Evaluation of Massage and Aromatherapy Massage in Palliative Care. 1998. In review for publication.

31. Interview with AMTA Foundation Grantee Pauline King. *Massage Therapy Journal*. 1997;36(1):117-120.

32. King, Pauline. Interview by author. Portland, OR. 3 March 1998.

33. Crawford, J. Myofascial Release Provides Symptomatic Relief from Chest Wall Tenderness Occasionally Seen Following Lumpectomy and Radiation in Breast Cancer Patients. *International Journal of Oncology, Biology, and Physics*. 1996;34(5): 1188-1189.

34. Brennan, M. and J. Weitz. Lymphedema 30 Years after Radical Mastectomy. *American Journal of Physical Medicine and Rehabilitation*. 1992;71(1):12-14.

35. Harris, R. An Introduction to Manual Lymph Drainage The Vodder Method. *Massage Therapy Journal*. 1992;31(1):55-66.

36. Manual Lymphatic Drainage Brochure

37. Weiselfish, S. An Interview with Bruno Chikly, MD. *PT and OT Today*. April 8, 1996. P. 12-13.

38. Hutzchenreuter, P.; H. Wittlinger; G. Wittlinger; and I. Kurz. Post Mastectomy Arm Lymphedema: Treated by Manual Lymph Drainage and Compression Bandage Therapy. *European Journal of Physical Medicine and Rehabilitation*. 1991;1(6).

39. Bunce, I.; B. Mirolo; J. Hennessy; L. Ward; and L. Jones. Post-Mastectomy Lymphedema Treatment and Measurement. *Medical Journal of Australia.* 1994;161:125-128. (7/18/94).

40. Zanolla, R.; C. Monzeglio; A. Balzarini; and G. Martino. Evaluation of the Results of Three Different Methods of Postmastectomy Lymphedema Treatment. *Journal of Surgical Oncology.* 1984;26:210-213.

41. Garnett, Karen. *What's New in the Prevention and Treatment of Lymphedema.* Cancer Rehab Conference. Portland, OR. Oct. 17, 1998.

42. Hornsby, R. The Use of Compression to Treat Lymphoedema. *Professional Nurse.* 1995; 11(2):127-128.

43 Field, D. and S. Miller. Cosmetic Breast Surgery. *American Family Physician.* 1992; 45:711-719

44. Heidt, P. Helping Patients to Rest: Clinical Studies in Therapeutic Touch. *Holistic Nursing Practice.* 1991;5(4):57-66.

45. Jurgens, A.; T. Meehan; and H.L. Wilson. Therapeutic Touch as a Nursing Intervention. *Holistic Nursing Practice.* 1987; 2(1):1-13.

46. Meehan, T. Therapeutic Touch and Postoperative Pain: A Rogerian Research Study. *Nursing Science Quarterly.* 1993;6(2):69-78.

47. Kramer, N. Comparison of Therapeutic Touch and Casual Touch in Stress Reduction of Hospitalized Children. *Pediatric Nursing.* 1990;16(5):483-485.

48. Wager, S. *A Doctor's Guide to Therapeutic Touch.* New York: Perigee Books/The Berkley Publishing Group. 1996.

49. Wetzel, W. Reiki Healing: A Physiologic Perspective. *Journal of Holistic Nursing.* 1989;7(1):47-54.

50. Barnett, L. and M. Chambers. *Reiki Energy Medicine.* Rochester, VT: Healing Arts Press, 1996.

51. Ray, B. *The 'Reiki' Factor in The Radiance Technique.* St. Petersburg, FL: Radiance Associates, 1992.

52. Pavek, R. *The Handbook of SHEN.* SHEN Therapy Institute. 1987.

53. Goodwin, J. Hospital Healer. *New Age Journal.* Nov/Dec 1996. P.47-56.

54. Knaster, M. Tiffany Field Provides Proof Positive Scientifically. *Massage Therapy Journal.* 1998; 37(1): 84-88.

Chapter 4

Piecing the Body Together:

Massage
for the Hospitalized Patient

When my mother started her nursing career fifty years ago, she performed nearly all of the care during a patient's hospital stay. Not only did she carry out typical nursing duties, but she was physical, occupational, and respiratory therapist all in one, as well as social worker, massage therapist, and housekeeper. Today, because of increased knowledge and technology, it is impossible for one health care provider to be all things to a patient. Modern-day care requires the use of a team comprised of many disciplines. All of the members of the patient's health care team, however, are working toward the same goals my mother had during her career.

Despite the many advantages of being cared for by specialists, there can be a down side to a dozen different staff members attending to their "piece" of the patient. The day consists of a steady stream of medical staff who briefly care for some part or another, leaving the patient feeling like Humpty Dumpty. The respiratory therapist cares for the lungs, the physical therapist sees to the legs, the nurse

I was frustrated today. It took me 1 and 1/2 hours to give a 15 minute massage. I went in and checked with the patient, Mr. B, but before I could get started, the doctor came in. After she left I returned, but the physical therapist came in. Soooo... I gave a massage to one of the nursing assistants, which she liked and appreciated. I went back to Mr. B and had just started working on his shoulder when the IV nurse came in. So, I gave Mrs. B a massage to her shoulders and neck. The IV nurse left and I was finally able to give Mr. B a little bit of massage to his feet.

— JENNIFER KRAMER, L.M.T.

manages the high tech machinery, the pharmacist is responsible for managing pain, the nursing assistant sees to the commode, the nutritionist oversees the food, the IV nurse attends to the central IV catheter, the social worker cares for the emotions, and the pastoral counselor attends to the soul.

Although unintended, this encounter can be de-personalized, invasive, and fragmenting. The body is often touched as if there were no one at home inside, or is associated with discomfort rather than pleasure. An unhurried session of light, comfort-oriented massage can be an antidote for the hospital experience. Attentive, loving touch can piece the body together again, as well as heart, mind, and soul, leaving the patient feeling "whole."

Massage in hospitals is not a new phenomenon. Before the onslaught of paperwork, nurses often gave patients nightly back rubs as part of getting them ready for going to sleep. Nurses are supportive of massage for their patients and many grieve at the turn health care has taken, putting them in the position of overseer and accountant, rather than that of true caregiver. A nurse, interviewed by Bill Moyers on the series "Healing and the Mind", related that she would never dare to stand by a patient's bed and hold her hand for fear of being caught. There are so many tasks to do that it would be considered a waste of time. Like art, music, and sports in the schools, massage is no longer seen as a necessity during a hospital stay, but as a luxury.

Giving massage in the hospital setting is often difficult for those who are trained as bodyworkers but have no other background in health care. By nature, massage therapists are sensitive, which is one of the things that makes them skillful, compassionate givers of touch. Yet this strength is also a weakness in settings such as hospitals, where the interventions are often invasive, toxic, or hurried. This sensitivity makes it difficult for some bodyworkers to adjust to working with the hospitalized patient because they feel so much of the stress, pain, and despair of patients, family, and staff. In order to be comfortable in the hospital, massage practitioners must come to grips with at least two paradoxes. The first, that of being simultaneously sensitive to the patient and insensitive toward the standard operating procedures inherent in a large health care facility. The second paradox is how we accept hospitals for what they are, and yet strive to make them more humane places to be. No easy solutions exist for these dilemmas. The immediate answer lies in the therapist's ability to embrace opposing energies, to hold both sides at once.

ADAPTING TO A NEW CULTURE

Massage can sometimes be given in the hospital as a simple, spontaneous act. I was able to do this for my father during a visit the day after his surgery. My visit coincided with the doctor's rounds, which allowed me the immediate opportunity to ask permission to massage my father's feet.

However, more often than not, performing bodywork in a hospital is analogous to traveling in a foreign land. Like people in a new culture, the staff in a hospital speak an unfamiliar language, have different habits, roles, and values, and dress to fit their environment and life-style. Travelers who adapt to the local "customs" find their journey is easier and more enriching when they "do as the Romans do." Bodyworkers who adjust to the expectations and protocols of the hospital culture will find their experience safer, more rewarding, and effortless.

LIABILITY

Concerns about liability influence the attitudes and behaviors of hospital workers. When practicing in the arena, massage therapists, too, must adopt a high level of awareness to it.

When a patient is hospitalized, that institution and its employees are responsible, or liable, for the care, treatment, and safety. Much of the treatment and care is performed by the nursing staff, physical therapists, occupational therapists, respiratory therapists, or nutritionists, but the physician decides on the overall medical and surgical treatment plan and writes the medical orders to be carried out. Nurses and other health care staff have no authority to prescribe drugs or medical treatment, unless further trained.

Generally, bodywork performed with hospitalized patients is for the purpose of comfort or relaxation and is not considered to be part of their treatment plan. Few health care institutions have massage therapists on staff to perform such a service, so most likely a bodyworker would be hired by the patient or family. In these cases a doctor's order may or may not be necessary. The patient's nurse will know the hospital's policy regarding doctor's orders for relaxation massage. However, if the patient desires bodywork to manage a specific symptom, such as lymphedema, it is necessary to obtain a doctor's order.

It is not unheard of for some bodyworkers, such as Reiki practitioners, to perform their modality with hospitalized patients without receiving permission first. Granted, many modalities are inherently safe, but the prudent thing for all bodyworkers to do is to check with the patient's doctor or nurse prior to initiating any work. Not only does this offer some liability protection, but also gives the practitioner a chance to interact with and educate the hospital staff about the benefits of the discipline. Even if it is a family member or friend who will be giving the massage, check in with the staff first.

No matter what type of bodywork is practiced, whether for relaxation or as a treatment measure, it is wise to carry a personal professional liability policy, especially if working on a fee for service basis. This is a requirement of many health care institutions. While the institution accepts major liability for patients' care, each licensed worker employed by the hospital is individually liable for performing his duties in accordance with the regulations and limitations of his licensing board or governing body. This is also true for practitioners who are not hospital employees, but come into the facility as independent contractors. On the other hand, bodyworkers who give massage as official hospital volunteers most likely would be covered by the institution's liability policy.

CONFIDENTIALITY

Hospital staff are legally and ethically obligated to keep information about a patient strictly confidential. So too are bodyworkers, whether working in the role as friend, family member, or professional. Those working in any health care setting must protect patient anonymity and confidentiality. Information regarding patients identity or why they are in the hospital cannot be revealed.[1] If there is a need to discuss an experience outside of the hospital, such as part of school clinical rounds, professional meetings, or in professional literature, omit using names or descriptions that might reveal a patient's identity, such as the diagnosis, age, date of admission, ethnicity, or name of the hospital. Rather than focusing on patients during an outside discussion, therapists should focus on their own experience.

Other examples of information that must remain privileged include discussions with or conversations overheard from other health care workers, information told by the patient, or knowledge gained from medical records.[1] Personal information about the patient should not be discussed among the health care team; only that which may be relevant to the patient's treatment or psychosocial well-being should be talked about.[2] Not only are professional touch therapists expected to follow these policies, but so too are those who offer their services on a voluntary basis.

Because of confidentiality, independent contractors, friends, and even family members wishing to give massage may or may not be given specific information from the nurse regarding a patient's status. For instance, if an independent contractor asks the nurse about the patient's platelet count, it probably would not be given out unless there is a physician's order. That data is available only to staff or official hospital volunteers. If specific information is desired, the practitioner must have the patient sign a release form. However, by asking three general questions, enough knowledge can be gathered to insure that the bodywork session will be performed safely even without exact patient data:

- Are there any conditions that demand extra light pressure?

- Are there any sites that should be avoided?

- Are there any position restrictions?

By and large, cancer patients are knowledgeable about their status and will fill in the information that the nurse may be unable to reveal for reasons of confidentiality.

Massage therapists must honor patients' rights to confidentiality, whether that patient is a friend, family member, or a client. However, a practitioner working as an independent contractor may be ethically bound at times to pass on knowledge that was originally intended to be private. If a patient's safety and well-being is in jeopardy, the bodyworker should report the situation to the patient's nurse or physician. For example, a bone marrow transplant patient commented during his massage that if he had it to do over again he would not have had the transplant. The experience had left him so tired and uncomfortable that he felt hopeless, wishing the ordeal to be over. Perhaps the nurse was aware of his feelings, but perhaps not. Patients will often say things within the relaxed atmosphere of a massage session that they won't say to other health care providers. By bringing the man's feelings to the nurse's attention, the nurse can assess whether more could be done to meet the patient's comfort needs.

If the patient shares information that should be discussed with the health care team, ask permission to do so. If refused, explain that it is being revealed for reasons of safety or to ensure well-being. These are the only reasons to break a confidentiality.[2] Massage therapists, however, who are on the hospital staff and are part of the patient's health care team, are expected to discuss all information that is relevant to patient care with their team members. Obtaining patient permission or informing them about the intent to share the information is unnecessary. However, within the context of the hospital and the health care team, confidentiality generally applies to data that is not relevant to patient care. For example, talking about a patient's political beliefs or sexual orientation among the staff would be irrelevant in most cases to the patient's care, and therefore a breach of confidentiality.

Rules of confidentiality are very clear-cut between professional health care providers and patients. But when massage is being given on a more informal basis to a friend or family member, the lines can become blurry, and facts that the patient preferred remain private can unknowingly be passed along to others within the social circle. It is acceptable to give out general information about the patient to other friends or family, such as, "She's not feeling well," or "He's very upbeat." However, no specific facts should be given unless the patient has consented. Examples of such precise information may include that the cancer has metastasized to the liver; that the patient is having trouble with his bowels; or that the cancer has gone into remission.

It is often tempting to call family and friends to announce changes in the patient's health status, but patients must be allowed to convey the specifics of their situation in their own way and time. An extreme example of violating a friend's privacy is the woman who put an announcement in the church bulletin of her friend's upcoming surgery for breast cancer. The patient, who was sitting in church on Sunday when the notice was read out, was horrified. Of course, the woman was only trying to be helpful, but she failed to understand that everyone has a unique feeling about their body and health status.

Some patients hold nothing back from friends or family. In those cases the bodyworker friend or family member might be more forthcoming about what they share with others if the patient has given permission. If the patient's preference for sharing information is not known, then the prudent and ethical course is to withhold anything that was communicated by the ill person, even to close family members. Patients will often tell things to a nurse or therapist that they would withhold from certain relatives.

Even though these regulations about privacy are explicit, learning to honor them requires diligent practice and is a process in which mistakes will be made. Americans have become a tell-all society, losing the reticence of previous generations. This openness has yielded many positive outcomes, but one negative effect has been a deterioration in peoples' ability to keep confidences.

HOSPITAL DYNAMICS

Bodyworkers often enter the hospital scene believing that the most difficult and challenging aspect will be in relating to people who are seriously ill. They may fear that the odors, tubes, machines, incisions, or wasted bodies will be overpowering. However, the most common angst comes not from the patients, but from the hospital itself. To the uninitiated, a hospital unit appears confusing and disorderly. Figuring out which of the multi-colored clad staff are nurses, doctors, students, physical therapists, or respiratory therapists is difficult. People new to the hospital scene often feel slighted when starting out because everyone just carries on with their duties with hardly a glance up. Rarely does anyone stop to assist the newcomer. Often students have said in seminar, "If they want us here, you'd think they would stop and be more helpful." This business as usual approach is taken as a snub, when it is the farthest thing from the truth. Nurses are thrilled for their patients to receive bodywork, but their work load is so staggering and stressful that there is little energy left over to give empathy to other health care team members.

Bodywork practitioners should expect to take the initiative in learning each hospital's routines, especially if they are volunteering or working independently. They may have to ask where is this, what to do with that, and how to get from here to there. Whether this is the best way to orient novices, or anyone else, is questionable, but it is a reality in today's rapid pace. It is up to the bodyworker to adapt to a particular area. Eventually rapport and trust will be established and the staff will begin to recognize the massage therapist as an individual, then as a member of the health care team they and the patients look forward to seeing. The bodyworker will literally be greeted with big smiles and open arms. But the transition from outsider to insider can be bumpy and long.

One of the most intimidating experiences is learning to get referrals from the staff or collect patient data from the nurse. Sometimes the practitioner must wait for the nurse to finish a task or series of tasks before she can speak to you. At other times it is appropriate to gently break into the current activity. Only experience will teach the novice when to wait and when to politely interrupt. To be sure, hospitals are not for the meek.

NURSING STAFF

The majority of staff interactions will be with the nursing personnel, which usually includes registered nurses (RN), licensed practical nurses (LPN), and certified nursing assistants (CNA). Regional differences exist in the use of nursing staff. In some states LPNs do not work in acute care settings, but usually will be found in long term care facilities. In the drive to cut costs, hospital administrations are moving toward less skilled and less costly employees. When this is the case, the nursing staff will be composed of a higher ratio of CNAs and LPNs. Because the care of oncology patients requires specialized skills, there are sometimes more RNs on these units.

It is the role of the RN to provide direct patient care, to oversee other auxiliary personnel such as CNAs, to coordinate the other health care practitioners, such as physical therapists or nutritionists, and to document the patient's condition. It is appropriate to ask for assistance from the RN (or LPN) in the following situations:

- To obtain pertinent patient data.
- To report changes in the patient's condition.
- To report colostomy bags or foley catheters that need attention.
- To report a problem with an IV or piece of medical machinery.
- To confer about unfamiliar skin conditions.
- To obtain help with any situation that is highly technical.
- To obtain assistance with linens or positioning a patient only if the CNA is unavailable.

The CNA assists the patient with the less technical tasks such as activities of daily living (ADL), positioning, lifting, transfers, vital signs, and basic charting. They may also assist the massage therapist in the following areas:

- Providing extra bedding, sheets, towels, or pillows.
- Positioning the patient.
- Assisting the patient onto the commode or to the bathroom.
- Changing sheets due to a bowel or bladder accident or vomiting.
- Removing a urinal, bed pan, or emesis (vomiting) basin.

rainbow
outside the patient's window,
nurses gathered at the doorway

— G. M.

Do not forget to cultivate a relationship with the housekeepers. They are often more than willing to take time to help with a variety of situations:

- Finding bedding

- Identifying staff members

- Taking care of spills on the floor, including broken glass (do not clean up yourself as body fluids may be involved).

One way to more quickly establish rapport is to offer some short, seated sessions to a few of the staff each time. This will help the staff to recognize the therapist as a person; it will acquaint them with the bodyworker's abilities, and help them to be more trustful to permit the massage therapist access to their patients. It also will give the practitioner a chance to educate staff about what their discipline offers to the hospitalized patient. Many RNs are unfamiliar with the wide range of touch modalities. Initially they may only refer patients from a selected few, not realizing that there is always a way to provide skilled, comforting touch if the patient so desires. By integrating some of the comfort-oriented techniques into the seated sessions, the staff will quickly come to understand that everyone is a potential candidate for massage.

Seated massage sessions for staff also give professional therapists a chance to market themselves. In addition, comfort and relaxation is provided for a group of very stressed health caregivers. Initially, both staff and patients were surveyed at OHSU before and after the massages. On the whole, the staff reported their stress to be greater than that reported by the patients.

SUGGESTED ATTIRE AND GROOMING

While hospital attire is no longer as rigid as it once was, the standards are more stringent than what is commonly worn in the bodywork community. Massage therapists will be more readily accepted if they attire themselves in a way that is appropriate to the standards of the institution.

- Shoes with closed toes and heels. This is a safety regulation set down by OHSA – Occupational Health and Safety Administration.

- Socks.

- Long pants or skirt that at least comes near to the knee.

- No shorts or mini-skirts, even in the summer.

- Shirt or blouse with a collar. In terms of being recognized it can help to wear a shirt of a color that is easy to identify. (OHSU volunteers wear purple polo shirts. The nurses have come to recognize the color immediately, which makes it easy for the volunteer therapist to gain access to the staff.)

- Do not use scents of any kind, such as perfume, cologne, or heavily scented laundry soaps, lotions, shampoos, or deodorants.

- Pull back long hair.

- No long, dangling earrings that could catch on the patient.

- Maintain short trimmed, clean nails.

STANDARD PRECAUTIONS AND PROTECTIVE ISOLATION PRECAUTIONS

All bodily fluids should be treated as if they are potentially infectious. Touch practitioners must protect themselves from body substances, which include blood, urine, feces, mucous, saliva, vomit, semen, and wound drainage. The steps taken to insure the safety of both patients and caregivers from bodily fluids are referred to as **standard precautions.**

Bodyworkers also can pose a risk to patients, especially cancer patients, who often have weakened immune systems. Actions such as handwashing, masking, and gloving may be taken to protect immunosuppressed patients from people with a communicable disease or exposure to one. These protocols are known as **protective isolation precautions**.

HANDWASHING

The hands are the most common way to pass contagion, making handwashing the most basic standard or protective isolation precaution. All bodyworkers are required to hand wash, even those who work through garments, such as Reiki Practitioners or Polarity Therapists. The hands and forearms should be washed just prior to beginning the session, after the patient data has been collected, the room arranged, and the bed adjusted. With patients who are severely immunocompromised, it will be necessary to hand wash prior to entering the room. There are generally instructions on the door if this is the case.

PROCEDURE:

1. Wet hands and forearms.

2. Use hot water at a temperature that is comfortable to you.

3. Soap hands and forearms, working soap into a lather.

4. Wash the entire surface of the hands (Figure 4-1.) and forearms for 15 seconds, including the fingers and under the fingernails. (Between patients it is necessary to wash only the hands.)

5. Do not touch the sides of the sink. If your hands accidently touch the sink, repeat the handwashing.

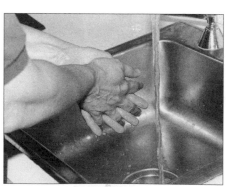

Figure 4-1.

6. Rinse well. Do not shake water off hands, as splashing spreads germs.

7. Dry with paper towel, then use the towel to turn off the faucet. This protects your hands from dirty faucets.[3] (Figure 4-2)

If you come into contact with body substances immediately wash the area with soap and water. Report the incident to the nurse. He will advise you on any further steps that should be taken.

GLOVING

Two types of gloves are available, vinyl and latex. Because oil stretches both types of glove, it is best to use lotion rather than oil. In most situations, vinyl is preferable to latex. The surface of a vinyl glove is smoother than that of a latex glove, which makes the massage experience more enjoyable. In addition, some patients and practitioners are allergic to latex. The symptoms can range from simple dermatitis to life-threatening anaphylactic shock. Although the latter outcome is highly unusual, less severe reactions to latex are becoming more common place. While latex gloves are less permeable than vinyl ones, studies have also shown that vinyl gloves offer a comparable degree of protection.

Always glove for the following situations:

•   To move a urinal, bed pan, or emesis basin that has been used. One glove is usually sufficient. Be sure to follow Step 2 under the removal procedures when taking off just one glove.

•   To touch any part of the patient where there is a possibility of contact with any body substances, including cuts or scabs.

•   If the therapist has a cut, open sore, scratch, abrasion, scab, or a non-contagious rash on the hands. (Do not give bodywork sessions with any kind of contagious rash, even with gloves. Wait until the condition has cleared.) A way to determine if an area is 'open' or 'intact' is to wipe the area in question with alcohol, if it stings, it is 'open' and should be covered with a glove.[4] If the scratch or sore is on the end of the finger, a finger cot can be worn to protect the area.

•   When any area of the patient's gown or linen is contaminated by body substances.

PROCEDURE FOR PUTTING ON:

1. Remove rings and bracelets to avoid puncturing or tearing the glove.

2. Wash hands and forearms.

3. Dry thoroughly. (Putting gloves onto damp hands can create skin problems.)

4. Put on gloves.

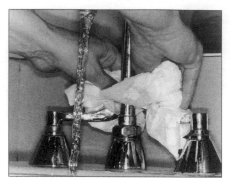

Figure 4-2.

REMOVAL: (FIGURES 4-3 AND 4-4)

1. Remove the first glove by grasping it with gloved hand in the palm and pulling off.

2. Remove the second glove by sliding a bare finger inside the glove and pulling up. Touch only the inside of the glove. Do not touch the outside of the glove with the ungloved hand. Fold the second glove over the first dirty glove as it is removed.

3. Place used gloves in a receptacle outside the patients room. Dispose of gloves after each use. Never re-use the gloves for another patient. Also, do not use a set of gloves for more than one activity, i.e., moving a full urinal, then touching a patient.

4. Wash hands thoroughly and dry.[3]

MASKING AND GLOVING

It is often necessary to glove and mask before entering the room of a patient who is immunosuppressed. There will be instructions on the door if this is the case.

PROCEDURE FOR PUTTING ON:

1. Apply mask

2. Wash and dry hands

3. Glove

REMOVAL: (REVERSE THE ABOVE PROCESS)

1. Take off gloves

2. Wash hands

3. Remove mask

GOWNING

Caregivers and visitors must occasionally gown when they are in the room of an immunosuppressed patient. This helps to protect the patient from microorganisms that may be on the clothes of those entering the room. Most gowns are disposable and for one use only; however, this may vary according to the hospital.

PROCEDURE FOR PUTTING ON GOWN:

1. Mask

2. Wash and dry hands

3. Put on gown without touching own clothing. Be certain it overlaps in the back so that all clothing is covered.

4. Wash and dry hands again without allowing anything to touch the gown or mask (i.e., sink or door).

5. Glove

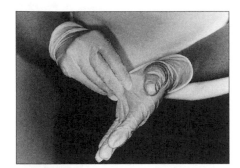

Figure 4-3.

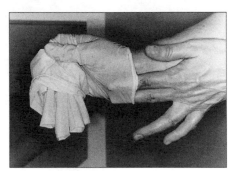

Figure 4-4.

REMOVAL OF GOWN:

1. Remove gloves as per procedure.

2. Untie waist and neck ties.

3. Remove gown by pulling off at the shoulder and folding inward and roll up into a ball.

4. Place in covered container.

5. Wash and dry hands.

6. Remove mask.

7. Wash and dry hands.[3]

LINEN HANDLING

It may be necessary to obtain additional sheets, towels, or blankets for draping, warmth, or to cover soiled areas. Linen is handled in many ways, depending on the facility. The recommended procedure is as follows:

1. Prior to collecting clean linen, wash and dry hands.

2. Remove the necessary items from the linen closet or cart.

3. Do not let linen touch your clothing.

4. If any linen falls onto the floor, discard it into the soiled linen hamper.

5. Consider any unused linen as dirty and place it in the hamper. Do not replace it in the closet.

6. When handling soiled linen do not let it touch your clothes.

7. When placing used linen in the hamper, simply place it in. Never plunge your hands and forearm down into the hamper to compact the soiled linen down.

8. Wash and dry hands.[3]

The patient's linen or gown may become contaminated by a variety of body substances, such as urine, feces, wound drainage, or blood. If a soiled area on the sheets is dried, a clean towel or draw sheet can be placed over that section to protect the touch practitioner. Ideally, linen that contains moist areas of contamination would be changed before starting the massage session. If it is not possible to have the sheets changed, wear gloves when working in the vicinity of soiled areas that are still moist. Placing a clean towel over these sections is not enough because the body substance will soak through. If the patient's gown is soiled by bodily fluids, either ask the nursing staff for a fresh one or wear gloves when working around the contaminated section.

HANDLING OF WORK CLOTHES

Granted, massage therapists do not often come into contact with bodily fluids, but it is prudent to get into the habit of handling hospital work clothes in the following manner. The shirt worn to the hospital should be clean, because this is the article of clothing that is most likely to come into contact with the patient. Since hospitalized cancer patients are commonly immunosuppressed, every precaution must be taken for their consideration.

- The shirt should always be put on clean just before departing for the hospital. Do not wear it to work with other clients or to do other sorts of work.

- If it is necessary to bring the clean shirt to change into, place the shirt in a container that is used only for that purpose. For instance, do not place the clean shirt in a backpack or athletic bag that is also used to carry the multitude of items we cart through life. A one-gallon Ziploc bag works nicely. Do not put a clean shirt in yesterday's dirty Ziploc.

- After finishing at the hospital, remove the work shirt. Do not wear it to another work site or around home. This protects those the touch therapist lives with, as well as other people who receive bodywork from her.

- Do not smoke and try to avoid smokers after putting on hospital clothes. Cancer patients are often highly sensitive to odors and can become nauseated in their presence.

THE MASSAGE SESSION

Finally, all of the preliminaries are over. The nurse has been contacted, the patient data obtained, hands washed, and materials gathered. The therapist can now get to the business at hand, being with the patient. This is the part that many novices think will be the most difficult, but it is the easiest and most rewarding part of the experience.

BEFORE THE SESSION

The massage begins the moment the therapist enters the room. Through her being the bodyworker projects comfort and relaxation. Movements should be calm, slow, and gentle when entering the room, moving hospital furniture, or doing intake. "Match your movements to the patient's energy level which is generally slower than the world outside the room."[1]

PRIOR TO TOUCHING THE PATIENT:

1. Hang out the "Massage in Session" sign. This doesn't guarantee you won't be interrupted, just that the intrusions might be made more gently.

Massage eases pain no longer through deep tissue or myofascial or range of motion techniques, but through understanding and support, communicated through the presence and undivided attention of professional touch...just placing gentle, attentive, caring hands on the patient is enough.

— PEGGY MAURO,
Massage Program Coordinator
Boulder Community Hospital

You're not only touching the body, but the individual. The agenda, if you were to have one, is to be with the patient, not to give a massage. Massage therapists may have to drop techniques in favor of just being there. It's amazing how putting our attention on someone can shift things.

— Dawn Nelson,
Compassionate Touch Workshop,
Oregon School of Massage,
March 1997

2. Discuss with the patient what she would like from the massage, taking into account any cautions regarding her condition.

3. Identify all IV sites, dressings, open areas, lesions, and sore, painful areas.

4. Arrange the room so there is a path around the bed. It will help the session to flow better if you don't have to stop in midstream to move furniture, IV stands, or stacks of newspapers.

5. Generally there will be sufficient pillows, linen, and bedding in the patient's room. If it is necessary to leave the room to obtain more blankets, towels, or pillows, be sure to re-wash before touching the patient.

6. Practitioners new to hospital work must let go of their expectations about establishing the perfect environment. Controlling all of the noise and chaos is impossible. However, it is possible to help the patient create an atmosphere more conducive to relaxation. Suggest that the television be turned down or off and the phone be unplugged if no calls are expected. Dim the lights if possible.

7. Raise the bed so that you can stand almost completely erect. Many bodyworkers are accustomed to setting their tables lower to gain leverage. Leverage is not needed here, as the desired outcome is usually a comfort-oriented session. Raising the bed will not only insure that the pressure is lighter, but it will also save the practitioner's back.

8. Close privacy curtain if applicable. If the patient shares a room with other patients, it is good to acknowledge the roommates before closing the privacy curtain to begin the session. "This supports privacy because when the roommates are acknowledged, included, and not ignored, they can more comfortably allow the patient and the massage therapist to be alone."[2]

9. Lower the bed rails. IV tubing, surgical drains, or catheters are often in the vicinity of the bed rails. Be very mindful when lowering or raising them so as not to catch the tubing.

10. If the patient needs help to position herself, ask the nursing staff for assistance.

11. After everything has been arranged and you are ready to begin, wash hands and forearms.

During the Session

1. When conversing with the patient, follow her lead. In general, these conversations are much like those you would have with anyone else. Topics such as children, pets, the garden, and occupations are common subjects of discussion.

Some patients openly talk about their illness, but many do not. Mostly, people want to be understood. The goal is not to "fix", but to appreciate what is happening. Talking with patients and family members is a dance—they lead, you follow.

2. Allow the patient to do as much for himself as he would like. In sessions with a healthier individual, the therapist might encourage him to completely relax and permit himself to be pampered. However, people who have been ill for a long period of time often feel guilty about the number of daily tasks that must be done for them. If the patient shows an interest in adjusting the bed or helping during draping, allow him to assist you in these ways.

3. If the session is interrupted by doctor's rounds, ask the patient and physicians if they would prefer you to leave, to wait on the periphery of the room, or to continue massaging.

4. Do not hesitate to ask the patient to move closer to the side of the bed if she is able. This will be much more comfortable for the therapist. If she is unable to move without minimal assistance or without causing pain, work with her where she is.

I massaged her as if she was a flower, or a piece of fine china. Those images helped me to stay soft.

— PAULA BENTLEY, L.M.T.

5. Drape in much the same way as when working with a client on a table. One of the main exceptions to this is surgical patients for whom any excessive movement may be painful. In those cases, simply lay the bedding gently aside without tucking it in. Hospital patients invariably lose much of their modesty after the myriad procedures where the body is exposed, but this does not mean normal draping procedures should be abandoned. Only expose the body part being massaged. An exception to this would be a patient who is overly warm and has been lying on top of the bed anyway.

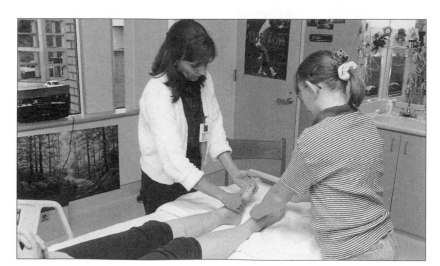

Figure 4-5.

Proceed with the massage, moving the gown aside when necessary. Often a cancer patient may have been in the hospital for weeks and prefers to wear personal clothing, such as a sweat suit. Undressing for a massage can be difficult because of IV tubes threaded into the arm or neck of the garment. It is often easier in these situations to administer bodywork through the clothing. (Figure 4-5.)

6. Check with the RN if any uncertainties arise, such as skin conditions. Remember that the hospital and RN have the primary responsibility for the patient's care and safety. Outside practitioners should not make unilateral decisions about conditions they feel they could treat. For instance, if the beginnings of a bed sore are found, there might be the temptation to address the problem with common Swedish Massage techniques. Before embarking on such a treatment, the nurse should be consulted.

7. If a nurse is needed immediately, step to the door and call for her. Pushing the call button may not get an immediate response.

AFTER THE SESSION

1. Wash hands briefly to remove lotion or oil.

2. Lower the bed and raise the bedside rails.

3. Replace the overbed table and telephone within reach.

4. Tidy the patient's bed.

5. If lotion or oil was used on the patient's feet, wipe them so that they are not slippery.

6. See if there is anything else the patient would like done before leaving.

7. Have closure with the patient. Consider each session a one-time window of opportunity to be with that person. It is natural to say, "See you next week." However, there may be no next week. The patient may be discharged unexpectedly, they may take a turn for the worse and be transferred to intensive care, or may die. Instead, you could say, "I enjoyed our time together," or wish them "All the best." Saying good-bye each time is important

8. Remove massage sign.

9. Thoroughly wash hands and forearms after leaving the patient's room.

It is best....to avoid repetitively asking, "How are you?" Although this is an innocent and often automatic question, it often makes the patient feel like a failure for not having improved. It is more helpful... to let the patient know that they enjoy his company, despite his disability.

— SUSAN WAGER, M.D.
A DOCTOR'S GUIDE TO THERAPEUTIC TOUCH

INDICATIONS FOR ADMINISTERING TOUCH

Because a way always can be found to give gentle, soothing touch to people with cancer, the term "indications" rather than "contraindications" is used here to more accurately reflect the possibilities. "Indications" is a positive word that creates confidence instead of fear. However, practitioners must massage carefully and mindfully. Working in this manner will produce confidence.

MAJOR ALERTS

Bodyworkers should be especially alert to three situations: 1) deep vein thrombosis (blood clots), 2) leukopenia or neutropenia (low white blood count), and 3) thrombocytopenia (low platelets). Touch can be administered to patients with these three conditions. However, each situation calls for special care with regard either to the modality used, the amount of pressure, or the need for observing strict protective isolation precautions.

DEEP VEIN THROMBOSIS (BLOOD CLOTS)

Deep vein thrombosis (DVT) is potentially very dangerous. A blood clot could break free as a result of some kinds of bodywork, and get stuck in a smaller vessel, blocking the flow of blood and oxygen to the tissue fed by that vessel. If one of these emboli (a blood clot that has broken free) gets stuck in the lungs, the consequence can be fatal. Bodywork should be performed only after receiving permission from the medical staff.

Those who are in danger of developing blood clots, such as post-surgical patients, often have a therapeutic wrap on their legs called a sequential compression device (SCD). (Figure 4-6) SCDs contain tubes that electronically inflate and deflate to maintain the circulation in the legs. This is to help minimize the chance of a deep vein thrombosis developing. Patients with a diagnosis of DVT will be on anticoagulants, such as heparin, warfarin, or even aspirin. Anticoagulants cause interference with the blood's ability to clot by inhibiting the production of fibrin. A delicate net that entangles red blood cells, white blood cells, and platelets is constructed from fibrin. These trapped cells can then become a clot.[5] Medical staff will usually approve massage once the blood has thinned to a certain level and stabilized.

Subtle energy techniques (S.E.T.s) have been used successfully in this situation. Modalities such as Reiki, Polarity Therapy, and Therapeutic Touch (TT) are examples of S.E.T.s. These disciplines work with an intangible energy in the body which is referred to as universal life force in Reiki, electrical energy in Polarity, or the human energy field (also known as the aura) in Therapeutic Touch. S.E.T.s are useful where pressure or increasing the circulation is

There is nothing stronger in the world than tenderness.

— HAN SUYIN

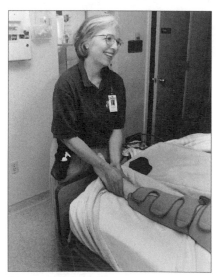

Figure 4-6.

contraindicated, as with DVT. With these techniques the hands rest on or above the body but no pressure is applied.

THROMBOCYTOPENIA (LOW PLATELETS)

Platelets are one of the components of blood that cause clotting. Typically, a cubic millimeter of blood contains 200,000–300,000 platelets.[5] However, when the numbers are insufficient, around 10,000–20,000, bruising occurs easily and clotting occurs slowly. The worst case scenario would be to cause internal bleeding, which once started is difficult to stop. However, this would not occur if bodywork is administered gently and carefully. Thrombocytopenia may be induced by certain drugs such as prednisone, chemotherapy, and radiation, and often accompanies leukemia, myeloma, and some lymphomas. Patients with low platelets often will be hesitant to accept massage during this time. However, light effleurage usually can be performed safely if the patient wishes to have bodywork. Occasionally the platelet level is so low that patients aren't allowed to brush their teeth for fear of bruising the gums. During these times only S.E.T.s should be administered. (Figure 4-7)

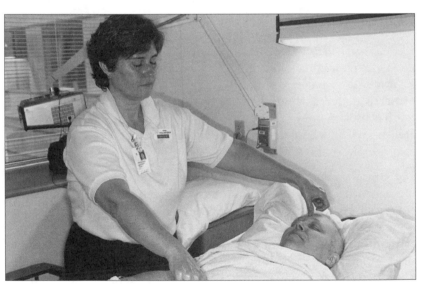

Figure 4-7.

Most nurses and physicians are unfamiliar with the broad range of bodywork modalities. Their knowledge may come from the experience of receiving massage as a healthy person or from information seen in the popular media where massage is given in a more vigorous manner. When approached about administering bodywork to their thrombocytopenic patient, they may initially have a lukewarm attitude toward the idea. The touch practitioner can help by using such phrases as "gentle massage" or "light touch" and briefly demonstrating light touch on the doctor's or nurse's back. This will give the medical staff a different frame of reference. Be certain to ask permission from the doctor or nurse before reaching out to demonstrate on their back.

It's best to "under-do" rather than "over-do" if a choice must be made.

*— KAREN GIBSON,
DEVELOPING A HOSPITAL-BASED
MASSAGE THERAPY PROGRAM*

A normal white count is between 4,300 and 10,800 leukocytes per cubic millimeter.[5] A low white count may be brought on by chemotherapy, radiation, drugs, or disease. The patient's immune system is suppressed leaving them especially vulnerable to contagious diseases such as herpes, the flu, or even bacteria from their own skin. Massage is indicated for these patients, but bodyworkers must remember to apply protective isolation precautions to all patients at all times. Most likely they will be required to perform longer hand washings, and, if the white count is severely low, may even need to mask and glove. At first it can be disconcerting to give bodywork while masked and gloved, but it gets easier each time. Massage lotions can be used with gloves (use lotion supplied by the hospital during this time) or you may prefer to use bodywork techniques such as light compression, Shiatsu, or S.E.T.s that don't require a gliding motion. Always hand wash immediately prior to touching the patient and after the room has been set up and the bed adjusted. The bodyworker should never work with an immunosuppressed patient if the practitioner has a cold, flu, fever, or any communicable illness. Neutropenic patients often don't feel well, so massage extra gently.

SURGICAL PATIENTS

Surgery is the most invasive form of cancer treatment. It may appear that the patient is completely in the hands of the surgeon and is dependent on them for a positive outcome. However, there are steps the patient can take to influence the surgical process. Many techniques, including massage, can be used to increase relaxation, which can help patients recover more quickly and have less pain.

PREOPERATIVE

The night before surgery is often anxiety-ridden. Massage can calm the patient and assist her to relax before going to sleep. Energy therapist Julie Motz likes to "lay her hand lightly over the area to be operated on. 'Just to relax that part of the body and make it feel loved, and prepare it for what is about to happen.'"[6] This is also an excellent time to incorporate guided imagery or mental rehearsal techniques regarding the next day's surgery.

DURING SURGERY

Giving energy work during surgery is still highly unusual. Julie Motz is pioneering its use in operating rooms at Columbia Presbyterian and Beth Israel Hospital in New York City. She has worked along side surgeons operating on patients for brain, breast, and pancreatic cancers. Both patients and operating room staff have found her presence to be calming. Patients are thought to recover more quickly from anesthesia and have less nausea and vomiting.[6]

... offering energy medicine to surgery patients prior to, during, and after surgery may provide greater comfort and relief of some common postoperative adverse effects. Not only does [energy medicine help] the patient heal more readily and without problems, but the entire medical setting seems to work more coherently and smoothly.

—JACLYN STEIN HENDERSON,
*THE POWER OF ATTUNEMENT
THERAPY:
STORIES AND PRACTICE*

POSTOPERATIVE (*FIGURE 4-8.*)

Gaining access to the operating room may prove to be difficult, but with a little planning and assertiveness, patients wishing to have a touch practitioner with them in the recovery room may have success when approaching their surgeon. Although there is no scientific evidence, anecdotes from subtle energy practitioners suggest that administering touch immediately after surgery may speed and ease the recovery room process.

Depending on the type and location of surgery, the patient may be able to have very light effleurage applied to the feet and hands soon after returning to the room. If this type of touch is contraindicated, subtle energy techniques may be used for the first few days. Pay special attention to the liver and kidneys by working the reflexology points on the feet or the associated acupressure meridians. Reiki can also be applied directly over the liver and kidneys. These organs are crucial to the body's eliminating toxins from drug and anesthetic agents. Obtain physician permission and guidance before initiating bodywork for postoperative patients.

INCISIONS

Bodywork on incisions is contraindicated for 4-6 weeks. When that time period is over, it is advisable to get physician approval prior to working the surgical area. The use of S.E.T.s 1-2" above incisions often provides some relief from the pain of the incision.

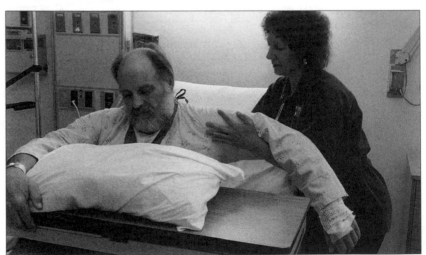

Figure 4-8.

ANTICOAGULANTS

Surgical patients may be on anticoagulants, such as heparin, coumadin, or aspirin, to dissolve blood clots, to prevent them, or to thin the blood. Bodywork should be done lightly, with broad strokes, as bruising occurs easily. Anticoagulants can cause a rash called petecchiae, which is characterized by very small red or purplish spots.

The spots are the result of blood leaking from blood vessels into the tissues. Light pressure over these areas is usually fine.

HICCUPS

To a patient with a fresh incision, the hiccups are more than a mild annoyance. Each of these bodily jerks may be excruciatingly painful. Slow, gentle massage to the feet can induce relaxation, and without the patient even realizing it, the hiccups are often relieved. A more pernicious form of hiccups can also be caused by irritation to the phrenic nerve due to a tumor, fluids from the tumor, or as a result of surgical manipulation in the abdominal area. Relieving these hiccups is extremely difficult, even with the use of drugs.

MEDICAL DEVICES

INTRAVENOUS/CENTRAL LINES

Two general types of intravenous devices will be encountered: 1) peripheral lines, which are inserted into the lower arm or the antecubital space (at the elbow joint). Only work below the site of a peripheral line, i.e., wrist and hand. Avoiding the area above the peripheral site insures that massage will not cause a surge in whatever is being administered through the IV, such as medications, blood products, or chemotherapy. It also insures that the IV will not be dislodged or that the patient will not be caused discomfort by the IV moving around. 2) The second type of intravenous device is the central line, which is usually surgically inserted into the chest. (Figure 4-9) This may be a "port", which lies just beneath the skin, or a line that exits externally. Discomfort may be caused, especially when lying prone, necessitating side-lying techniques when working on the back.

Parents at her bedside,
Poison dripping through the tubes,
The fight begins.

Beautiful daughter lying there,
Hard to see her with no hair,
Fear fills the room.

Through her fear she smiles,
Through her pain she smiles,
Hope remains.

— JULIE McDOWELL, L.M.T.

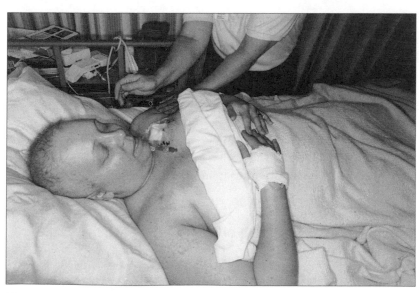

Figure 4-9.

Another type of central line may be inserted into the antecubital space of the arm. These central lines are referred to as peripherally inserted central catheters (PICCs). Central lines are left in for long periods at a time; patients then do not have to be "stuck" over and over again by needles. The central line contains an opening (lumen) through which the nurse can give medications, chemo, electrolytes, etc. Do not work in the area of a central line. With a PICC only work the hand and wrist. There may be bluish bruises around any IV site due to the trauma of inserting the IV or reddish streaks caused by irritation from the drugs given during chemotherapy. Never massage these areas.

FOLEY CATHETER

A Foley is a urinary catheter. After the catheter has been inserted into the bladder, a small balloon at the end of the tube is inflated with sterile water to keep the catheter in place until it is removed. The patient may not want to lie on the abdomen while the catheter is in. S.E.T.s rather than Swedish Massage are indicated in the abdominal area so as not to interfere with the catheter.

NASOGASTRIC (NG) TUBE

NG tubes are inserted into the nose and extend into the stomach. They are used to administer nutrients and liquids or to empty fluids and gases from the stomach. It is not uncommon for the throat to be extremely irritated by the tube. S.E.T.s have often been found to reduce the throat irritation to a tolerable level. The practitioner's hands do not touch the throat, but are held an inch or two above for at least 5–10 minutes.

COLOSTOMY OR ILEOSTOMY

A colostomy is an artificial opening of some part of the colon onto the abdominal surface. An ileostomy is the same procedure performed on the ileum, which is the lower 60 percent of the small intestine.[5] Usually these procedures are needed after a section of the colon or small intestine has been removed. A pouch is placed over the opening (stoma) to collect the intestinal contents. The new colostomy and ileostomy bags are lightweight and inconspicuous. Most colostamates use disposable pouches that are kept in place by a face plate that adheres to abdomen.[7] Stool from a colostomy is usually soft and formed while stool from an ileostomy is liquid.

Not all colostomies or ileostomies are permanent. Sometimes after the bowel has healed, the two ends of the bowel can be rejoined, or "taken down", to use medical terminology.[7] Whatever the case, bodywork can still be administered to the remainder of the body. Some people will prefer to leave their underwear on during the massage and may not want to lie prone. A side-lying position can be used to massage the back.

John's right kidney had been removed and he hadn't been able to urinate since. He had meditated about the removed kidney, but had not been able to shift into a place that felt healing. Reiki, he hoped, would get things "flowing" again. After only a 30 minute session, the Reiki effortlessly shifted him. He reported that the empty spot where the kidney had been filled with energy, and a body-wide flow of energy was re-established. Now he felt as if he could move on to healing himself. Once again he was balanced. I also gave Reiki just above the incision. He reported that during the session the discomfort caused by the incision, NG tube, and IVs were completely forgotten. Prior to the session he rated his comfort at a 4 (5 is extremely uncomfortable). Afterward he rated his comfort at a 1 (extremely comfortable).

— G.M.

If the patient wishes, there is usually no physical reason to avoid touching the abdominal area. Some people have physical pain at the colostomy site, others don't. Receiving massage in this area can help the patient become more at ease with the situation. As with any other situation, universal precautions need to be followed when working in the area around the colostomy.

MEDICAL PROCEDURES

Touch can be calming and reassuring to a patient undergoing almost any medical or nursing procedure, such as stem cell collection (Figure 4-10.), having a new IV inserted or an old one attended to, or during an arterial puncture. Simply holding the head, feet, or hands is often sufficient to relax patients during this time. Following these procedures, the sites may benefit from the application of subtle energy techniques over but not touching the site. Wait until all tenderness has vanished before applying pressure to the areas. Bodywork can also be beneficial during a magnetic resonance imaging (MRI) test for the patient who is claustrophobic, or while receiving chemotherapy.

BONE MARROW TRANSPLANTS

Today, the term bone marrow transplant (BMT) often means a stem cell transplant. Stem cells, which are found primarily in the marrow, are primitive blood cells that grow into red blood cells, white blood cells, and platelets. Some stem cells also circulate in the blood, but their numbers are not sufficient for a full transplant, necessitating the use of some bone marrow cells.[8]

Part way into the massage an IV nurse came in to replace and flush out the patient's central line. I chose to remain in the room during the procedure. While the nurse worked I stood behind the patient with my hands on her shoulders. When the procedure started, I could physically feel what was going on with the patient. It was a feeling of pain at the heart and nausea. The nurse checked with the patient, who verbally described these sensations. The nurse also asked if she could feel the love that was coming from me through my hands. The patient answered that what she felt was strength. I had to leave the room for a minute to recompose myself, but was able to continue the massage OK after that.

— KIRSTI, L.M.T.

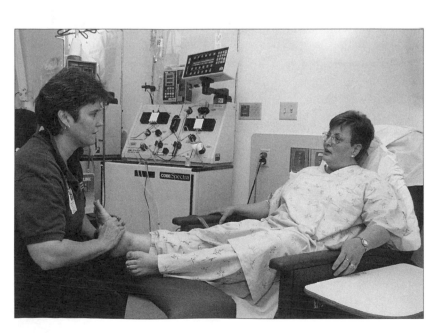

Figure 4-10.

Bone marrow transplantation is sometimes involved with certain cancers, such as breast cancer, lymphoma, leukemia, and myeloma (bone marrow cancer). This procedure allows the use of chemotherapy and radiation doses three to ten times the ordinary dose. These high dose treatments kill not only the cancerous cells but also destroy components vital to the blood and immune system: red blood cells necessary for oxygen transport, white blood cells needed to fight infection, and platelets used for clotting blood. Bone marrow transplantation attempts to counter the destructive effects of the chemotherapy and radiation used to treat cancer by rebuilding the blood and immune systems.[9]

The bone marrow or stem cells are infused through the patient's central line, which then find their way back to the bone marrow where they will grow and produce new healthy blood cells. Patients whose stem cells are collected from the blood generally recover in two weeks, leaving them able to fight off infections more quickly. This may be due to the stem cells in the blood already being more mature, requiring less time to complete their development. The recovery of patients whose stem cells are taken from the marrow often takes five weeks, increasing the period they are at risk from infection.[8]

There are two types of bone marrow transplants, autologous, which is the most common, and allogeneic. In an autologous bone marrow transplant the patients donate their own marrow prior to undergoing high doses of chemotherapy and/or radiation, while in an allogeneic transplant bone marrow is given by another donor whose marrow is a genetic match.[9] Those receiving their own marrow recover more quickly and have fewer side effects. People who receive marrow from another person take much longer to recover and may have side effects that last for years. These patients must develop a new immune system, making them more susceptible to any infection than a normal individual. This is especially true during the first 100 days after transplant, but remains true even after several years. As with other immunosuppressed cancer patients, practitioners should avoid working with these patients if the practitioner is ill. This is critical during the first 100 days when the transplant recipient's immune system is fragile or non-existent. A simple infection from a microorganism that is benign to a healthy person can be lethal to a patient in this weakened state.

The high doses of chemotherapy given with this procedure cause agonizing side effects, such as high fever, nausea, vomiting, painful skin rashes, mouth and esophegeal sores, and severe fatigue. Thrombocytopenia is also common with chemotherapy and requires extremely gentle pressure. Patients who have donated their own bone marrow will have an aspiration site, usually at the hip. These sites should be avoided, as they are sore for about a week.

GERI

Geri was a 45 year old woman with acute lymphocytic leukemia who could have been my big sister. She had dark hair mixed with gray, cut really short in back. Her face was broad at the top and ridged with lines. When I went into her room to introduce myself, Geri's pain was evident from the lines on her face. She sounded vague and shaky from the morphine given in preparation for a bone marrow biopsy. Geri knew from three previous aspirations how painful the procedure can be and was extremely frightened. She and I agreed on a plan to massage her legs, which were achy, and I promised to stay and hold her hand while the doctor did the bone marrow aspiration.

Geri was moaning and was frantic with pain. Her nurse, Nancy, gave more pain killer through the IV while I started to massage her feet and legs in an effort to soothe her, but almost immediately, two doctors came in to get the patient's permission to do the procedure. She signed the papers and also spoke of her anxiety over the pain.

The doctor asked Geri to roll onto her stomach in order to find a spot on her sacrum to do the aspiration. Her sacrum and lower back were badly bruised and the puncture wounds from the previous three procedures were obvious. Both doctors pressed over these bruises to feel the sacrum to either side of the spine, causing Geri to cry out from pain. She lost control and started sobbing. Through all of this I was doing my best to be unobtrusive and give her some physical comfort.

The doctors chose a spot, stressed to Geri that she must lie still during the procedure, and told Nancy to administer more pain killer. When they left for a few moments, I moved up to the head of the bed and began giving Reiki to Geri. The doctors were soon back, along with a technician who had the tools for the aspiration. Nancy gave another round of analgesia. When that dose took effect, there was a big change in the patient. Her face grew slack and her limbs were limp. Five shots, all painful despite the pain killers she'd already had, were then given to anesthetize the skin, tissue, and bone at the site. Geri's anxiety was so intense she felt everything despite the staff's attempt to make her comfortable. I was sure someone would send me away, but no one paid me any heed, so I kept on stroking her back, neck, and head.

The procedure was difficult to watch. The doctor used a thick, four inch needle with a handle of sorts on one end. After swabbing the area with betadine solution, he pushed the needle down to the bone, and screwed it into the sacrum. Geri's back hyperextended from the force, sinking into the mattress. Blood ran freely from the puncture. Off and on she would moan and cry out. I held her left hand and stroked her hair. Everyone in the room was tense. Nancy asked to give more morphine; the doctors agreed.

The first needle was removed and another longer thicker biopsy needle was inserted down to the bone. I didn't watch. With each twist and push of the needle I could feel Geri's body jerk. After several attempts, a tiny amount of bone marrow was extracted. By then I was feeling numb from controlling my reactions. As the doctors finished up their work, I closed the Reiki session and left.

Now, 30 hours later, I am amazed at my ability to remain calm through such an incredible experience. I'm glad that I hardly knew this woman. Even now I feel her fear and pain and worry about how she is doing. I hope Geri felt my touch and knew that someone was holding her hand and stroking her face. It isn't important that she knew about me, just that she felt the presence of someone sympathetic who could share her pain.

— *Jacqueline McCal, L.M.T.*

Eventually neutropenia will occur, which requires strict adherence to protective isolation precautions. Anyone who is ill or has a fever, flu, or cold must not visit a BMT patient during this time. Remember to use lotion supplied by the hospital during periods of immuno-suppression – lotion in bottles brought from the outside may contain potentially harmful germs. Also, when visiting a BMT patient do not bring gifts that may harbor bacteria or fungi, such as fresh fruits, vegetables, and fresh or dried flowers.[10]

Patients who receive allogeneic transplants are afflicted by additional side effects referred to as graft versus host disease (GVHD). GVHD occurs because the new bone marrow (the graft) sees the body (the host) as an enemy and attacks it. This is the opposite of an organ transplant in which the body sees the new organ as the villain and tries to reject it. GVHD most often affects the skin, gastrointestinal tract, and liver, resulting in skin rashes or discoloration, nausea, vomiting, and diarrhea, liver dysfunction and jaundice.[11] With the exception of skin rashes, none of these symptoms precludes the patient from receiving a session of gentle touch.

ISOLATION

Patients with severely suppressed immune systems, such as those who have had a BMT, will often be placed in a special unit or in an isolation room for protection. (Figure 4-11.) The air pressure in these rooms is adjusted so that when the inside door is opened, the air in the room exerts an outward, pushing force, thereby keeping outside air from the patient's room. In the past it was thought to be necessary to completely isolate these patients and no one was allowed in the room. Today, healthy family members, friends, and hospital staff come and go freely, but with a lot of lengthy handwashing. Masking, gloving, and even gowning are precautions also commonly taken before entering an isolation room. If these precautions are necessary, they will be conspicuously posted on the door. Working the first time in these rooms can be unnerving. The massage therapist fears she will pass on germs that to her are completely benign, but to the patient can be deadly.

Now I know what the hands of an angel feel like.

— FRANK,
BONE MARROW TRANSPLANT PATIENT

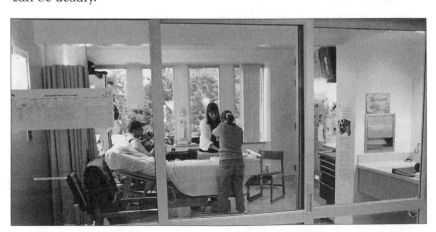

Figure 4-11.

SIDE EFFECTS FROM TREATMENT

ALOPECIA (LOSS OF HAIR)

Chemo patients lose their hair because the chemotherapy is toxic to hair cells on the scalp. The shaft becomes brittle, causing the hair to break off. There is no reason to avoid touching the head unless the patient is uncomfortable with it. Having the head touched in a loving way can help the patient to accept himself. (Figure 4-12)

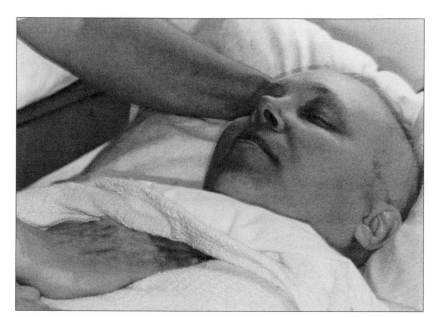

Figure 4-12.

BREATHING DIFFICULTY

Fear and anxiety can bring on a variety of breathing problems, such as shortness of breath, rapid breathing, or contraction of the throat and bronchial tubes. Touch is extremely helpful during these episodes. Something as simple as holding the patient's feet or head can relax the breath.

CONSTIPATION

This is one of the most excruciating side effects of pain medications and chemotherapy. It is not uncommon for cancer patients to be admitted to the hospital because their bowel stops moving. During this time the patient's abdomen may be so painful that only light touch with no stroking can be tolerated. S.E.T.s can sometimes help the bowels to move or at least take the edge off the discomfort. However, many times the pain is nearly intolerable and nothing short of radical treatment will resolve the problem.

ANNIE and BILL

Annie was in the hospital because the various medications she was taking weren't interacting well. In addition, the chemo used for throat cancer left Annie severely constipated. On a scale of 0-10, with 10 being severe, Annie rated her pain at a 9. When Kendra and I offered her a massage, Annie said she didn't think she could, due to a lack of mobility. Her abdomen was painful from gas and blocked bowels, and a central IV catheter prevented her from lying face down. We explained there was no need for moving or turning in bed, that we could massage whatever was accessible without her moving. Annie agreed to this.

While Kendra began the session with Annie, I asked her husband, Bill, if he would like a shoulder massage. He declined, so I left to see another patient. Ten minutes later Kendra tracked me down to say Bill had changed his mind and would like a seated massage. His wife didn't want him to leave the room, so Bill and I worked in the corner, quietly discussing people we both knew and our common Scottish ancestry.

Kendra, meanwhile, was applying newly learned Polarity Therapy techniques to the painful areas of Annie's abdomen. The Polarity quickly started movement in the bowel. Peristaltic activity increased, gurgling sounds started, and Annie burped several times. Bill questioned Kendra about what he could do to help his wife relax. She talked to him about breathing techniques, meditation, guided imagery, and the effectiveness of simple touch. Together they each held one of Annie's feet for several minutes. Kendra then showed him ways to position his hands on his wife's head.

Following the session Annie's pain had dropped to a 3. But best of all, she had a bowel movement ten minutes after the bodywork ended.

— G. M.

EDEMA

Edema in the cancer patient is caused by a complex set of factors, such as nutrition, renal dysfunction, inactivity, and tumor growth. If the patient wishes to have comfort-oriented massage applied to a limb that is edematous, the following four guidelines should be employed: 1) Elevate it, either using pillows, as with the arm, or by raising the foot of the bed for the legs; 2) Use a light effleurage or light rhythmical compressions with the palm massaging towards the heart; 3) Begin massaging at the most proximal section of the limb (the upper arm or thigh), then move down to the next section (the forearm or lower leg), and then do the hand or foot. Massaging in this sequence allows the area "upstream" to empty, thereby creating space for the fluid that will drain from the lower regions. 4) Give attention to the joints, as fluid pools there. If the bodyworker is familiar with passive range of motion (ROM) exercises, these could be used to assist the movement of fluid through the elbow. Check with the nurse before initiating ROM exercises.

These guidelines are intended for use only with common edema situations resulting from not being ambulatory or as a side effect from chemotherapy. Therapists wishing to work with patients who have more serious, chronic lymphedema problems, such as those that accompany breast cancer, should be formally trained in one of the lymphatic drainage techniques. Always obtain a doctor's order to perform this type of bodywork.

NAUSEA

A quiet session of bodywork can help diminish nausea which is often a side effect of cancer treatment. Patients who have already received bodywork and know the process are very likely to want this gentle touching, knowing that the soothing effects will help with the nausea. Those who have never had bodywork will most likely decline, thinking that any extra movement will add to their discomfort. For some patients who don't feel well, being touched seems too much to bear. As always the decision must be left to the patient. Nauseated patients may have an emesis basin by their side and may even need to stop to use it during the session. If it is necessary to move the basin at any time, use universal precaution protocols and glove the hand that will be in contact with the basin. This will protect the practitioner from coming into contact with any infectious agents as well as any potentially toxic chemicals. The chemicals used in chemotherapy are very toxic and remain in the body and body fluids for up to 48 hours after completion. After removing the gloves wash your hands before resuming with the patient.

I was so amazed at how well massage transfers into the hospital setting. I think the reason I felt like crying after giving tonight's session was because of the sacredness of my encounter with massage in the hospital and the depth at which my patient and I met.

— ELIZABETH THORPE, L.M.T.

RADIATION BURNS

Patients with radiation burns are often passed over as appropriate massage referrals until the nursing staff realize that a well-rounded bodyworker will be skilled in some modality that can provide nurturing touch to these people who are even more touch starved than the average patient. Initially, the practitioner may have to use an off-the-body technique such as Therapeutic Touch. But eventually a modality such as Reiki or Polarity Therapy can be introduced. Avoid techniques that apply pressure or movement if the skin is fragile or broken. It is imperative to check with the nurse before using lotion on skin that has radiation burns. If the patient prefers not to have the irradiated areas touched in any way, massage the feet and hands and any other unaffected areas.

SHINGLES, HERPES, AND CHICKENPOX

These three diseases are caused by the same family of viruses and are a serious event to someone with cancer. Varicella, the virus responsible for shingles and chickenpox, can disseminate to the liver, spleen, central nervous system, GI tract, bone marrow, and lymph nodes. Shingles, a close cousin of chickenpox, and herpes are viruses that remain dormant in the body and become reactivated during times of immunosuppression, such as occur to people with cancer.[12]

Bodywork should never be performed in an area affected with vesicles, as each of these lesions contain a fluid which is highly contagious. Avoiding these areas will protect the practitioner and prevent further spread of the virus on the patient's body. If there is any doubt about which areas have been affected, always glove. Because the eruptions occur predominantly on the torso, the safest course of action is to give massage on the extremities until the skin lesions have dried and the scabs have disappeared. A patient with shingles can cause chickenpox in others who have not previously been infected.[12] Therefore, bodyworkers who have not had chickenpox should not administer touch to infected patients to reduce the possibility of contracting the virus and spreading it to other patients.

SKIN

A variety of skin problems are created by radiation, chemotherapy, and medications: dryness, rashes, burns, hive-like wheals, poor wound healing, disrupted integrity, breaks, hyper-sensitivity, severe itching, and lesions. Always obtain information from the nurse about any sites that should be avoided. Massaging with lotion is very helpful for people with dry skin, but with most of the other conditions listed is contraindicated. One exception is petecchiae, a rash with reddish purple dots. It can be gently massaged using lotion. Lotion can also be used on skin that has become paper thin, but it should be applied with the utmost care to avoid causing tears.

Additional information is given in the next chapter regarding chemotherapy, radiation, medications, and bone metastases. This knowledge is also relevant for working with people in the hospital.

*I put my hands on
your body. I felt your soul.
You/ me/ hands/ flesh/ soul.*

— JACQUELINE McCAL, L.M.T.

AUDREY

When I went in to ask if Audrey would like a massage, she cheerfully declined, saying she was fine and to give the massage to someone who needed it. "Should I come back if I can't find enough 'takers'?" I asked. She immediately said, "yes", and reached for her shoulders. "They get really tight from knitting." Audrey seemed to want a massage, but didn't want to be a burden. By presenting the opportunity in such a way as to make feel her she was doing me a favor, she could accept it.

Audrey was 64 years old and undergoing chemotherapy for bladder cancer. She was in the hospital to receive an infusion of red blood cells to combat severe anemia. Audrey had a peripheral IV line in her left arm and a urostomy bag on the right side of the abdomen to collect urine. Her bladder had been removed several weeks before. At the age of 12 her right kidney had been removed, leaving a deep crevice.

The session began with the intention of massaging her "knitting" muscles for 15 minutes. I thought if the opportunity presented itself, I would suggest extending the time. Because of the urostomy on her right side, she was only able to lie on her left side. I pulled the covers down to the top of her hips and untied the strings at the back of the gown to have access to her back and neck. I began by resting one hand at the base of her neck and the other on the upper sacrum, allowing us both to quiet. I asked her to let her eyes close and bring her attention to her breath. After several minutes I lightly applied massage lotion and gently gave effleurage to the back, shoulders, upper right arm, and neck.

Audrey had lost her hair from chemo and wore a bright blue turban with fake bangs. As I began to massage the base of the occiput, she admitted to being shy about people seeing her stubbly head. However, without my asking, she pulled the turban up a little to give me greater access. I ended the massage on her back with a Polarity hand position, one hand on the crown chakra, the lower hand on the sacrum. Before touching the top of her head I asked permission because of the shyness she had expressed.

When Audrey returned to her back, I asked if she would like some attention to her feet. She was more than agreeable. In order to have skin-to-skin contact with her feet, I pulled the tightly tucked sheet and blanket out from the foot of the mattress. Part way through massaging Audrey's feet, her roommate returned from a stroll around the halls. I stepped to the side and held Audrey's near foot in both hands while nurse, patient, and IV stand threaded their way through the obstacle course in the cramped room.

The session ended with light compressions up the legs to a final Polarity position, one hand on the crown chakra, the other on the heart chakra. When I left, Audrey was lying hands and arms thrown back, resting on the pillow above her head, all sense of imposition gone.

— G. M.

FINAL THOUGHTS

Cancer is a disease characterized by too much growth too fast. Registered Nurse Cheryl Chapman describes it as a "heat syndrome."[13] In addition, the nervous system is overloaded from pain, medications[14], and the excessive stimulation of medical staff in and out of the room. Massage sessions should aim to calm, cool, and slow, allowing the patient to rest and heal. Practitioners must shift their attention from muscles to skin, from effort to ease, and from stimulating to soothing.

The day shift in a hospital is anything but soothing and restful. Bodywork sessions are often cut short, interrupted, late in starting, or are unable to be scheduled at all because of lab tests, physical therapy, pastoral visits, or consultations with the doctor. Whenever possible, evenings are the best time for patients to receive massage. Not only are there fewer intrusions, but it helps the patient to relax before going to sleep. Although patients tend to have more visitors in the evening, this can be viewed as an opportunity rather than as an interruption. More and more, I try to teach family and friends how to give attentive touch by having them work with me for part of the session.

A patient once commented after her massage that it was a pleasure to have an interaction with a beginning, middle, and end. Usually, she explained, her encounters felt more like punches or stabs. People lunged in and out to administer drugs, deliver food trays, or consult about discharge plans. The massage session smoothed over the frayed ends created by these inevitable but necessary interactions. "I feel put back together again," she offered. Present-day circumstances require a team of practitioners to care for each patient. Hopefully, the time will come when skilled touch is once again seen as a necessity and every team includes a massage therapist.

TOUCH MODALITIES APPROPRIATE FOR HOSPITAL USE

Techniques that can be administered with little or no modification:

Attunement Therapy®   Jin Shin Jyutsu®

Bowen Technique   Polarity Therapy

Compassionate Touch®   Reiki

Cranialsacral Therapies   Therapeutic Touch

Bodymind modalities that incorporate touch with awareness techniques, dialogue, and emotional release:

Hakomi   SHEN

Rosen Method®   Somatoemotional Release®

Rubenfeld Synergy Method®   Somatosynthesis

Bodywork modalities that may be performed using gentle pressure:

Acupressure   Reflexology

Esalen Massage   Shiatsu

Jin Shin Do®   Swedish Massage

Kripalu Bodywork   Trigger Point Therapy

The Glossary of Bodywork Techniques in the Appendices gives a brief description of each modality. Not every modality is appropriate for every patient. For instance, some of the last group of techniques would not be safe for a person with extremely low platelets, but could be used with other patients. When I am in doubt about the amount of pressure to apply, I ask the nurse if I could demonstrate various pressures on her.

REFERENCES

1. Dunn, T. and M. Williams. *Massage Therapy Guidelines for Hospital and Home Care*. San Francisco: Planetree, 1996.

2. Dunn T.; X. Geiser; S.O. Cormier; J. Wagner; and L. Koch. Confidentiality in the Hospital. *Hospital-Based Massage Newsletter*. 1997; 3(2):18-28.

3. Graves, L.; L. Mullen; and J. Fouts. *Nursing Assistant Training Manual*. Medical Express, Beaverton, Oregon, 1992.

4. Dodge, J. Universal Precautions. *Hospital-Based Massage Newsletter*. 1997; 3(3):9-13.

5. Thomas, C.L., ed. *Taber's Cyclopedic Medical Dictionary*. Philadelphia: F.A. Davis Co., 1993.

6. Goodwin, J. Hospital Healer. *New Age Journal*. Nov/Dec 1996. p.47-56.

7. Booklet titled *Colostomy: A Guide*. American Cancer Society. 1991.

8. Antman, K. When are Bone Marrow Transplants Considered? *Scientific American*. 1996;275(3):124-125.

9. Booklet titled *Bone Marrow Transplantation: Questions and Answers*. Leukemia Society of America. 1991.

10. *Oregon Health Sciences University Bone Marrow Transplant Unit Guide for Visitors*.

11. Randolph, S.R. Home Care of the Bone Marrow Transplant Recipient. *Home Healthcare Nurse*. 1993;11(1): 24-28.

12. Ellerhorst-Ryan, J.M. Infection in *Cancer Nursing: Principles and Practices*. Boston: Jones and Bartlett, 1993.

13. AMTA National Convention Report. *Massage Therapy Journal*. 1997;36(1):82-95.

14. Mauro, P. and L. Koch. Specific Techniques for Specific Ailments. *Hospital-Based Massage Newsletter*. 1996;2(3):4-5.

Chapter 5

Reclaiming the Body:

Bodywork for People Living with Cancer

The experience of cancer shatters the self-image and traumatizes the body, making patients afraid and distrustful of their own body. It feels as if it is no longer theirs, belonging instead to a doctor who directs what will be done to it. Cancer also weakens the sense of hope and separates body from mind and spirit. Touch can help in restoring all of these areas in patients' lives, reminding them that the body can still be a source of pleasure, and that they are lovable despite being bald from chemotherapy, disfigured from surgery, or edematous from prednisone. It gives them hope that if their body can respond so positively from a one hour massage session, there is potential for healing. A massage helps in reclaiming the body and reuniting it with heart, mind, and soul.

[Milton Trager] knew that the essence of his work was reaching people's souls through their physiology.

— MIRKA KNASTER

When a massage client receives a cancer diagnosis it does not mean bodywork must stop, nor does it mean that a person with cancer cannot start receiving massage. In fact, loving, compassionate touch is needed all the more. Bodywork sessions can continue through every form of treatment, before and after surgery, and during chemotherapy or radiation.

People with cancer want to be touched, but sometimes are afraid friends and family will be repelled. Family and friends are similarly affected by this dilemma. They incorrectly assume their loved one does not want to be touched because of changes in her body. Sandy, an RN who nursed bone marrow transplant patients, noticed when she became sick from cancer her friends stopped hugging her. And yet this was the time she most needed their physical closeness and reassurance that despite a "big, hideous face and body" she was still lovable. Massage can be one way family, friends, and bodywork practitioners can give patients the touch they need.

The focus of this chapter is on those who are no longer hospitalized but are in the process of learning to live with or are recovering from cancer. This includes those who are recuperating from surgery, those still receiving chemotherapy or radiation, those whose cancer is being managed as a chronic illness, or those in remission. These patients may still be on medications, may be affected by permanent or semi-permanent medical devices such as central IV lines or colostomy bags, or may have permanent damage to nerve tissue in the hands or feet. However, a way can be found to touch all of these people.

MASSAGE DURING TREATMENT

The therapies used for cancer are often used in conjunction with each other, such as surgery and radiation for breast cancer or chemotherapy and radiation with bone marrow transplantation. These treatments can be employed as curative, rehabilitative, or palliative measures. When used as curative agents, surgery, radiation, and chemotherapy are attempting to eradicate the cancer. However, a cure is not always possible, in which case the goal is to use palliative measures to control the cancer and improve the quality of life. For instance, surgery, radiation, or chemotherapies may be used to remove or reduce the size of a tumor that is causing pain or obstructing a vital organ. Palliative surgery may be performed in the case of a large tumor that is impinging on other organs. It also may be used to prevent the development of a serious problem, such as obstruction of the superior vena cava or the collapse of a vertebra due to spinal metastases. Surgery also is performed for rehabilitative reasons, such as breast or facial reconstruction, skin grafts following resections for melanoma,[1] or the fashioning of a neobladder out of the lower portion of the bowel after surgery to remove the bladder.

Palliative treatment is offered primarily to relieve distress from symptoms, as well as for the patient's emotional well-being. Continuing chemotherapy or radiation, despite the progression of the disease, helps some people remain hopeful, which in itself can be enough to increase the quality and length of life.[1] Taking an active role in the process is important to patient's outcomes. In "Massage

Therapy and Persons Living with Cancer," Annette Chamness writes that patients who "take charge of their lives... empower all the forms of healing they participate in, from traditional Western medical treatments, to visualization, diet, acupuncture, exercise, and even massage therapy. They also have hope."[2]

As with hospitalized patients, the goals when giving massage to those still in treatment should be comfort, relaxation, distraction, or as an expression of intimacy and affection. Only gentle, loving touch should be performed when a person is undergoing treatment because of the side effects caused by each of the treatment methods. The skin is drastically affected by many of the therapies, such as medications, chemotherapy, and radiation. Many patients are susceptible to easy bruising as a result of drugs, low platelets, or fragile veins. During bouts of nausea and diarrhea the patient feels agitated and unsettled and wants to be soothed and calmed rather than stirred up. In addition, the patient's body is already flooded with toxins from chemotherapy. Deeper bodywork would add to the toxin load, further burdening the circulatory and immune systems. Refer to the chart in the previous chapter for bodywork modalities that are appropriate to give during the treatment phase.

Bodyworkers may work with these clients in the office, an outpatient clinic, or the client's home. Appointments may need to be scheduled to avoid times of peak nausea and diarrhea or immunosuppression. When the immune system is suppressed there may be times the client cannot be in public and the bodyworker will need to make a house call. If the therapist is the slightest bit unwell she should avoid being around the immunosuppressed client. Never expose an immunosuppressed person to illness. Every time a client with cancer comes for a massage, check the health status. Dramatic changes can occur in a short period of time when the person is in the treatment phase.

When first beginning to massage people with cancer it is important to err on the side of caution. Doing too little is preferable to doing too much. The practitioner should work within his comfort level. If a client asks for massage around a certain site or pressure that the therapist is uncertain about, he should gently refuse and stay within his comfort zone. People recovering from cancer need to be touched with calm, confident, and loving hands. Undoubtedly, giving massage while in a state of fear will affect the quality of the session. It is important therapists be able to fully embrace the person with cancer and be comfortable with the massage treatment plan they have developed. When questions arise from a session, the bodyworker should seek out guidance afterward from someone familiar with cancer patients, such as a nurse, another touch practitioner, or a physical therapist.

Without a doubt it is necessary to take special care when giving bodywork during the treatment phase. Practitioners must remain vigilant about the pressure, the client's comfort, and any sites that must be avoided. However, any energy used to maintain this extra

Esther is a perfect example of the power inherent in taking charge and having hope. Five months after being diagnosed with pancreatic cancer, which often causes death within several months, she started weekly Reiki sessions. Esther lived another year. She felt the Reiki sessions prolonged her life, but I think she survived mostly from the hope generated by pursuing potential treatments. The day Esther lost hope was apparent; she arrived for her Reiki session greatly fatigued and dispirited, the sparkle gone from her eyes. That morning her doctor told Esther nothing else could be done, that she was wasting her time to continue searching. Esther never recovered after the hope had been taken away.

— G.M

mindfulness is worth the effort. Therapists who work with cancer clients are repaid tenfold by the appreciation and gratitude shown.

SURGERY

If desired, gentle bodywork can begin as soon as the patient is home. Before administering bodywork that increases the circulation to post surgical patients, obtain physician approval. The risk of a blood clot, or thrombus, developing that could occlude a major artery, especially in the leg, is always a possibility following surgery because of the increase in clotting factors. (Carcinomas are also thought to activate clotting factors,[3] which puts some patients with these types of cancer at risk for developing a thrombus with or without surgery.) Depending on the patient's medical history and type of surgery, the physician might approve Swedish Massage the day after surgery. The most prudent course of action may be to use subtle energy techniques (S.E.T.s) for the first few days so that the circulation is not increased in case a clot has developed. A patient is unlikely to be discharged from the hospital with deep vein thrombosis (DVT) until definitive treatment has been started. However, it is not always possible for medical staff to discern the presence of a deep vein thrombosis because the condition sometimes occurs without signs or symptoms. Practitioners must be mindful of the influences that put a person at high risk for DVT. Besides increased clotting factors, there are two other main causes of deep vein thrombosis: venous stasis, which can be caused by general anesthesia during surgery or lack of movement following surgery, and damage to blood vessel walls.[3]

An extremity affected by deep vein thrombosis may exhibit any of the following four symptoms: 1) cold to the touch; 2) lack of sensation; 3) whitish or bluish discoloration; and 4) no pulse below the obstructed site. If any of these symptoms exist, modalities that increase the circulation, such as Swedish Massage, should not be administered to any part of the body. Do not palpate the area and immediately notify the doctor. If a clot has occurred, the patient will be put on anticoagulants and immobilized until the clot dissolves on its own. Following treatment for a blood clot, always get permission from the doctor to administer Swedish Massage.

Because the direction in health care is toward more outpatient procedures and shorter hospital stays, surgery patients are not allowed to linger in the hospital any longer than necessary. Women are often discharged one day after a mastectomy, a colon cancer patient can be sent home a day or two after having part of the bowel removed, or a man who has had a prostatectomy can be discharged in a similar amount of time. This trend means a greater reliance on home care, requiring family and friends to deal with drains, dressings, colostomies, feeding tubes, and catheters. It is necessary to determine the location of any medical devices before starting the session to avoid displacing them.

Scarring, adhesions, and lymphedema are potential side effects from surgery that can cause both localized and general problems. Pain, decreased range of motion, and loss of function can happen from each of these conditions. On top of this, secondary problems occur when patients "guard" these injured areas, causing them to compensate with other parts of the body. Misalignments then occur in the body as a whole, triggering new regions of discomfort in distant places. Many bodywork modalities can improve or resolve these three surgical side effects. Aston-Patterning, Myofascial Release, Neuromuscular Therapy, and Trigger Point Therapy are some of the techniques that can be helpful when massaging adhesions or scars.

ELEANOR

Bodyworker Beth M. has found Aston-Patterning to be beneficial for cancer patients following surgery. One 52 year-old client, Eleanor, came to her six months after a lumpectomy, removal of two-thirds of the lymph nodes, and chemotherapy for breast cancer. The client had severe pain in the affected arm, adhesions, poor mobility, and had become alienated from that part of her body. Aston-Patterning (AP), best known as a method of movement re-education, also contains fitness and bodywork components. Beth employed an AP technique known as myokinetics to release the adhesions in Eleanor's chest wall and arm and a movement education technique called neurokinetics was used in conjunction with arm movements to expand the client's breath. By the end of two sessions Eleanor was able to perform more weight bearing exercise, was better able to function in her Yoga for Cancer Survivors class, and felt more confident and positive about her body. The bodywork played an important part in these outcomes, but equally valuable was the education the practitioner gave to her client. Beth was able to help Eleanor understand what had occurred in her body as a result of the cancer treatments. Because of this knowledge Eleanor was able to relax into her recovery process, knowing that the body, with assistance, could eventually heal.

A variety of lymph drainage techniques are useful for clients with lymphedema or an impaired lymphatic system. Four groups of cancer patients are at a higher risk for damage to the lymphatic system: 1) women who have had a lumpectomy or mastectomy, even with no visible edema in the arm or hand; 2) men who have had a prostatectomy, even with no visible edema in the legs; 3) patients with edema in the extremities or trunk; and 4) patients who have undergone lymph node dissection or radiation.[4] Massage practitioners must be cautious not to apply too much pressure to areas affected by lymphedema or in cases in which the lymphatic system may be impaired. Superficial lymphatic vessels can be damaged from the compression of deep or even moderate strokes, such as are applied in Swedish Massage. Dr. Vodder, the originator of Manual Lymphatic Drainage, recommended that tissues be handled very gently, like a "cat's paw".[5]

Wait at least two months after treatment has ended and the oncologist has declared the patient in remission to initiate modalities that are more invasive or treatment oriented. This gives the cells and tissue time to recover without interrupting the rebuilding process. In the meantime, administer a technique such as Reiki or apply pressure to the acu-points along the meridians connected to the surgical area. Practitioners should study these methods with experienced instructors before using them with clients who have cancer. It is not the intent of this book to offer instruction in any modalities.

Brief descriptions of common surgeries are found in Appendix A. Other information regarding surgical patients is found in the previous chapter.

A note about people with skin cancer: These patients, even those with malignant melanoma, should be approached exactly like all others who have undergone surgery or other treatment for cancer. Skin lesions should not be massaged, mainly because it causes discomfort. However, the remainder of the body can be massaged appropriate to the stage of treatment or recovery. The American Academy of Dermatology (1-888-462-DERM ext. 22) publishes a pamphlet with colored photographs that can help bodyworkers recognize potential skin cancers. The pamphlet is titled "Skin Cancer: An Undeclared Epidemic."

DRUG TREATMENTS

In addition to the drugs given to kill cancer cells, patients are prescribed many other medications to address the side effects of treatment or the disease. Many of these drugs have a minimal effect on the massage process, others clearly impact it.

CHEMOTHERAPY

In the broadest perspective, chemotherapies are any drugs used to treat illness. In oncology, the term "chemotherapy" refers to drugs given to kill, slow, or stop the growth of cancer cells. Different antitumor drugs and different combinations of drugs are used for each type of cancer and work by various means. Most chemotherapies affect the cells' DNA, interfering with cell reproduction; others change the hormonal environment.[6] These drugs are designed to attack tumor cells which reproduce and grow very rapidly. While the intended target is tumor cells, other fast growing cells get caught in the cross fire, such as those of the skin, hair, nails, the lining of the digestive tract and blood cells in the bone marrow. The results can be the loss of hair, skin with rashes or tears, nausea and vomiting, anemia, and immunosuppression.[7]

Rather than being a reason to stop bodywork sessions, chemotherapy may indeed be justification for continuing and perhaps even increasing the frequency of sessions. When the fatigue and nausea are at the worst, patients frequently entertain the idea of stopping chemotherapy to get relief from their symptoms. Any intervention that can modify or alleviate these discomforts may help patients complete their treatment. As the research by Scott et al.[8] showed, a relaxation program that includes massage, given before and after chemotherapy, reduced nausea, vomiting, and diarrhea. Gentle bodywork can even be administered during chemotherapy. Patients spend endless hours in the outpatient clinic, waiting for drugs to drip into veins, waiting to see the doctor, or waiting for lab results. If nothing else, massaging hands, feet, and legs provides a pleasant distraction for patients and family. (Figures 5-1 and 5-2.)

The list of drugs used to treat cancer is extensive. However, many have similar side effects which are salient to the touch practitioner. These may include:

- Skin and hair: Dryness, sensitive to touch some days, breaks in skin, petecchiae (red or purple dots under the skin) and loss of hair.[9] Certain drugs given intravenously will cause a darkening along the vein. These darkened areas will usually disappear a few months after treatment has ended. People who have had radiation may develop "radiation recall" during chemotherapy. Some drugs cause the irradiated skin to turn red and may itch or burn. This reaction usually lasts from hours to days. Placing a cool, wet compress over the area may alleviate the symptoms.[7]

- Blood: Low platelets, low white blood count, anemia, fragile veins, easy bruising, and nosebleeds.

- G.I. tract: Nausea, vomiting, diarrhea, loss of appetite, and weight loss.

- Musculoskeletal system: Fatigue, malaise, weakness that can be debilitating.[9]

- Nervous system: Neuropathy in hands and feet due to the nature of the drugs. Patient may have burning sensation, intermittent shock-like pain, a sensation of "pins and needles," a "crawling" feeling, or tingling of skin or extremities. Other symptoms include poor balance, clumsiness, walking problems, jaw pain, and hearing loss.[7]

- Pyschoemotional: Depression, confusion, decreased cognitive skills, crying, emotional mood swings, and feelings of hopelessness.

- General symptoms: Edema due to hormonal changes related to the therapy or as an effect of the drugs.

Many patients on chemotherapy will have a central IV catheter, also known as a central line. Most often central lines are on the right side of the chest. The tubing is inserted into the large vein which leads into the superior vena cava. These types of central lines, which may also be referred to by their creators' names, such as Hickman, Groshong, or Quinton, protrude from the body and have several inches of tubing that extend out from an opening in the chest wall.

Another type of central line is a port-a-cath. This line, which has a port or reservoir, is inserted under the skin of the chest wall and has no external openings. The practitioner may see a slightly raised area

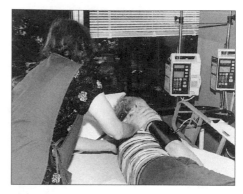

Figure 5-1.

This [massage] was wonderful. My body feels alive and I am in touch with it again. When she was doing my left hand it felt like I was getting a new hand.

— ROBERT, 41 YEAR OLD PATIENT WITH BRAIN CANCER

where the port has been placed. When touched, the area has a firm, hard feeling. Sites that contain either type of central line should be avoided during bodywork.

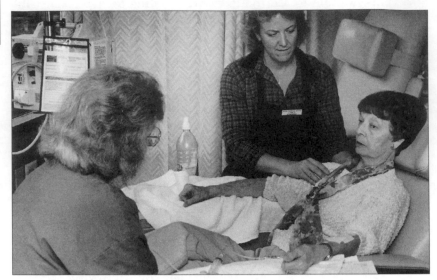

Figure 5-2.

Generally antitumor drugs are eliminated through urine and feces; therefore, skin-to-skin contact poses no threat to massage therapists. However, two of these drugs, **thiotepa**[10], also known as thioplex, and **cyclophosphamide**[11,12], also known as cytoxan, neosar, or procytox, have been proven to exit the body via sweat. Although the risk is minimal, it is prudent to glove when providing Swedish Massage or any other modality in which there is skin-to-skin contact to a patient who has received either of these drugs within the last 24 hours, including the time of infusion. It must be remembered that contact with the body fluids of all patients, including those undergoing chemotherapy, are to be avoided. Practitioners must glove if they are in a situation where contact with body fluids is possible, such as while moving an emesis basin or urinal.

Other drugs used in chemotherapy cause the pigment in the patient's skin to change color several weeks afterward. Usually the pigmentation changes occur in the face, palms of the hands, and soles of the feet. These changes are possibly due to an effect on melanin, the pigment that gives skin its color. This discoloration is in no way dangerous to bodyworkers.

Those who have undergone bone marrow or stem cell transplantation to combat the dangerous side effects of high dose chemotherapy may continue to be affected by the symptoms associated with graft vs. host disease (GVHD). Patients who have received their own stem cells, an autologous transplant, usually will not have the serious, ongoing complications of people who received marrow donated by another (an allogeneic transplant). Allogeneic transplants often continue to be affected by the symptoms of graft versus host disease (GVHD) for years. Each person manifests GVHD

I had expected the heavy-handed, "chop chop" massage seen in the movies. I was pleasantly surprised to receive such light, supportive touch.

— Karen,
+200 days since a bone
marrow transplant

in a unique way, but the common side effects are skin rashes, mouth sores which can extend down the digestive tract, and diarrhea, nausea, and vomiting. Swedish Massage should not be performed on skin that has a rash. Substitute an S.E.T. until the skin clears. These patients are commonly on prednisone and have low platelets, which precludes the use of deep bodywork.

People who have received stem cells from another donor must build a new immune system. Until the immune system recovers and all types of blood cells are being produced, patients are more susceptible to communicable diseases than the average person. The massage therapist with a cold or flu, or who has been exposed to other contagious diseases, should notify the client prior to their appointment so that the date can be re-scheduled.

(See Chapter 4 for other information regarding bone marrow and stem cell transplants.)

NANCY

Chemotherapy was a nightmare for Nancy the first time around. She suffered from nausea, diarrhea, fatigue, sleeplessness, drastic hair and weight loss, and was unable to work. When the breast cancer reoccurred a few years later, she sought out Reiki treatments in hopes of easing the side effects of the chemotherapy regimen. Nancy's plan was to go for chemotherapy after work on Thursday and spend the next three days recovering in time to return to work on Monday.

Reiki Master Phil Morgan would arrive at Nancy's house every Thursday at 5:30 just as she was coming home from the outpatient clinic. Nancy would lie down on the bed and within 30 minutes of starting the session she was asleep. Phil always gave special attention to the liver, kidneys, thymus, and adrenals. Two hours later he would quietly let himself out. Nancy would sleep through most of Friday and Saturday, wake up late Sunday morning and spend the day puttering around the house. By Monday morning she was ready for work. The Reiki sessions reduced or alleviated all of the side effects that plagued her the first time. Even the hair loss was much less.

The power of these hands-on treatments was made clear one week when Phil had to leave town and was unable to find a replacement. When she arrived home on Thursday evening after the chemo appointment, Nancy went to bed as usual, but could not sleep. The entire weekend she was nauseous and unable to rest. For the first time, Nancy was unable to go to work on Monday morning. Needless to say, she and Phil never missed another session.

It has been seven years since that round of chemotherapy and Nancy is still cancer free.

STEROIDS

The most common steroid drug prescribed to cancer patients is prednisone. This drug can be given in a variety of situations, as part of a chemotherapy protocol, as a pain medication, to elevate mood, or to increase appetite. Prednisone is often responsible for creating the round face that people with cancer acquire. Long term use of or large doses of prednisone have many side effects which have implications for bodywork. These may include:

- Skin: Can become parchment-like, wounds heal poorly, petecchiae, flushed, sweaty.

- Bones: Prednisone causes calcium to be leached from bones. High dose or long term use can cause osteoporosis. These patients may have hip and knee replacements more often than normal and fractures occur more easily.

- Blood: Low platelets.

- GI Tract: Diarrhea, nausea, and abdominal distention.

- Cardiovascular: More susceptible to hypertension, thrombophlebitis, embolisms, and tachycardia.[9]

- Psychoemotional: Mood changes, euphoria, and depression are common; high doses may cause delirium.

- General symptoms: Immunosuppression; edema – resulting from water retention. Light massage may be helpful in such an instance to get excess fluids circulating if kidney and cardiac function is adequate and fluid and electrolytes are stable.

NARCOTICS

Morphine is one narcotic commonly used to manage severe pain. Others may also include percodan, oxycodone, hydromorphone, and codeine. One of the side effects of narcotics is the depression of physiological functions. Side effects that may relate to massage are:

- Skin: Can be effected with rashes, easy bruising, flushing, hive-like wheals, profuse sweating, and itching.

- GI Tract: Can cause nausea, vomiting, cramps, and constipation. Constipation is the result of decreased peristalsis in the bowel.

- Cardiovascular: Can lower heart rate and cause blood pressure changes.

- Nervous system: Drowsiness, dizziness, confusion, or euphoria.[9]

ANTICOAGULANTS

The purpose of anticoagulants is to thin the blood and help prevent or dissolve clots. Patients with cancer are put on these drugs if they have a history of blood clots or to prevent coagulation problems. During hospitalization heparin is the drug generally given at first and then changed to warfarin. Outpatients are commonly prescribed warfarin or coumadin, which is a type of warfarin. The side effects of these drugs relevant to massage are:

- Skin: Rashes, wheals, easy bruising, severe itching, petecchiae.

- Blood: Low platelets, bleeding gums, blood in urine or stool, bleeding which is difficult to stop.

- GI Tract: Diarrhea, nausea, vomiting, cramps.[9]

ANTIDEPRESSANTS

Antidepressants are given to cancer patients for a variety of treatment purposes. Because depression is quite common and can amplify the perception of pain, by reducing depression, pain also may be lessened or better tolerated. These drugs also help to control a variety of other discomforts, such as insomnia and the tingling or burning pain from nerve injury. Amitriptyline and imipramine are two antidepressants commonly prescribed for people with cancer.[13] As with other forms of treatment, these drugs can cause side effects that may include:

- Skin: Rashes, wheals, itching.

- Blood: Low platelets and white count.

- GI Tract: Diarrhea, nausea, vomiting, cramps, constipation.

- Cardiovascular: Orthostatic hypotension (causes dizziness when standing up too quickly), tachycardia, hypertension, palpitations.

- Nervous system: Drowsiness, dizziness, confusion, anxiety, tremors, stimulation.[9]

RADIATION

Radiation is used to shrink tumors, to kill cancer cells, or to keep them from growing and dividing.[14] It accomplishes this by damaging the DNA in tumor cells. Usually radiation is given externally direct to the tumor site or to areas where the cancer might have spread. Full-body radiation may be given to treat cancers such as leukemia and lymphoma. When given externally, the radiation does not cause the body to become radioactive. Touching these patients is completely safe.

Radiation also is given internally, usually via an implant, which allows a more concentrated dose to be delivered at a specific site. Patients often will be hospitalized while receiving this treatment, but not always. Implants can remain in from a few days to six weeks. During long-term treatment with implants, the patient commonly remains at home and must follow special precautions to avoid unduly exposing others to the radiation. Because an area of the body is temporarily radioactive from the implant, giving massage during this time is risky to the practitioner and should be avoided.

Radioactive iodine is another form of internal radiation. Patients take this treatment orally and are radioactive for 48 hours. Bodywork can administered after the radioactive period is completed.

As with chemotherapy, normal cells are also affected, but the effects are most often related only to the area being treated. Besides fatigue, nausea, and diarrhea, the most noticeable effect of radiation is to the skin in the treated area. The skin may become very dry and look red, irritated, sunburned, or tanned. Usually the skin will recover several weeks after treatments end. In the mean time, treat it with the utmost tenderness. In some people the treated skin remains permanently darker.[15]

Touch therapists should adhere to the following guidelines when working with a client who is undergoing external radiation:

- Avoid massaging treated areas with strokes that use pressure or movement. At the most use only a gentle, still touch or work off the body if the skin is too irritated to touch.

- Prior to using lotion or oil on areas receiving radiation, check with the patient or the medical staff at the radiation oncology clinic. Many types of lubricants are contraindicated during this time because they can leave a coating that interferes with radiation and intensifies its effects to the skin. Some also interfere with the skin's healing, such as lotions that contain alcohol or metals. Alcohol dries the skin, and metals, such as zinc oxide or aluminum stearate, can cause rashes to skin that is tender from radiation. Even lubricants specially prepared for radiation patients can create skin problems because of certain ingredients, such as alcohol. Pure aloe vera gel, which rehydrates the skin and decreases inflammation, has been proven to be universally safe and beneficial.

  There also may be restrictions about applying skin products within a certain number of hours prior to the treatment. Practices differ from clinic to clinic. If the patient is unfamiliar with the exact guidelines regarding the use of lotions and oils, the practitioner should contact the clinic. The nurses will be knowledgeable in this area. Even if the clinic staff requests that no lubricants be used, massage can be administered over the clothing using Shiatsu, S.E.T.s, light compression, petrissage, or trigger point therapy.

- Do not use hot or cold packs on treated areas.

Radiation can also lower white blood cell counts and platelet levels. Low platelets are always an indication for gentle touch so as not to cause bruising. A low white count means the client is more susceptible to infection. The practitioner must take care not to work with the client if the practitioner has a cold, flu, fever, or has been exposed to other communicable diseases.

Deborah was diagnosed with breast cancer in 1994. Ever since, she has been on the incomprehensible roller coaster of remission – reoccurrence – remission – reoccurrence. Now, with metastatic lesions on her brain, she is once again undergoing radiation and chemotherapy. Prior to our first session together, she felt as if every cell in her body hurt. Following our second session she said she had previously rewarded herself after a radiation or chemotherapy treatment with the very best treat she could imagine, a Baskin and Robbins double rich chocolate malt. The best reward she now can imagine is her 45 minute massage. I hope I can continue to provide her with those brief moments of "time-out" from disease.

*— L.C.,
L.M.T.*

Note: Several massage therapists have reported that after massaging a patient on the same day the patient received external radiation, the therapist felt an intense and uncomfortable heat in the arms. Because radiation passes through the recipient and does not remain in the body, it is impossible for the reaction to have been caused by lingering radiation. Perhaps these practitioners were sensitive to the radiation on an energetic level. The majority of bodyworkers, however, can perform massage on patients who have just received radiation without consequences. The few who discover they are extra sensitive should wait until the following day.

Bone Metastases

Certain primary tumors tend to create secondary lesions in the bones and spine. The most common are breast, lung, kidney, prostate, and thyroid cancers. Other cancers that may metastasize to the bones are stomach, colon, pancreatic, and testicular. Bone metastases can cause decreased range of motion, a dull, aching bone pain, tenderness and warmth over the lesion, and are vulnerable to breaking. Rods will sometimes be inserted into the bone to stabilize it.[16]

Discerning between the pain caused by bone metastases and that by sore muscles is difficult for bodyworkers and clients. For example, a man sought help from a massage therapist thinking that the pain in his rib cage was muscular in origin. The ache, however, would not go away. The man eventually went to his doctor, where he was diagnosed with lung cancer that had metastasized to the ribs. Another man, who knew he had prostate cancer, sought massage to get relief from lower back discomfort. Because prostate cancer can spread to the spine and bones, the practitioner contacted the patient's oncologist to rule out bone metastases as the source of pain.

In general it is best to refrain from massaging these sites or work with extreme care. Many patients are able to tolerate some pressure and get benefit from gentle massage in the area. But for many, the area is so painful that even light touch is unbearable. A modality such as Therapeutic Touch, which is applied above the site, may have a soothing effect. As always, stay up to date with the progress of the disease by consulting with the patient's health care team.

Bodywork Following Recent Remission

Patients whose disease has recently been declared in remission should be slowly eased back to a more normal pressure over a number of sessions. Cancer treatments place a heavy toxin load on the body, which massage helps in eliminating. However, too much too fast may be more than the client's body can comfortably handle.

Bodywork modalities that use deep pressure, such as Myofascial Release, Rolfing, or Neuromuscular Therapy should be used only after the patient's oncologist has given the "all clear". There is no set guideline as to how long to wait after the patient has been declared cancer free. In his study using Myofascial Release with breast cancer patients, Dr. John Crawford waited eight weeks after treatment ended to administer MFR to his clients.[17] The clinic at the Rolf Institute has a policy of waiting 18 months after complete remission. Deep bodywork is intense and would direct energy away from the healing process.

If a client is still in treatment, has just finished, or is in recent remission, the following questions will assist the practitioner in gathering the information necessary for determining the correct course of action:

1. When were you diagnosed? What type of cancer was it? Where was it located?

2. What is the present status of your cancer? When was the last time you saw the M.D. regarding the cancer?

3. Are you being treated now? How? If not, when did you finish treatment?

4. Are there any sites restrictions because of:
   A. incisions
   B. skin problems
   C. medical devices
   D. tumor
   E. a recent history of blood clots
   F. bone metastases or a history of fractures

5. Do you have any pressure restrictions because of:
   A. anticoagulant medication
   B. a low platelet count
   C. neuropathy in the hands or feet
   D. steroidal medications
   E. osteoporosis
   F. bone metastases
   G. areas of fragile or sensitive skin

6. Do you have any position restrictions because of:
   A. tumor
   B. medical devices
   C. incisions
   D. tender skin due to radiation

If it is necessary to contact a client's physician to discuss health conditions, bodyworkers should obtain the client's permission in writing. When speaking to the doctor the therapist should: 1) describe the goals and the general treatment plan for the sessions; 2) explain the benefits of massage for that client; and 3) inquire about precautions.[18] There is no consensus among the medical community or the bodywork community about when to have a written doctor's prescription and when to allow a verbal order. In my opinion, a written permission should be required only when the client is known to have active cancer or when the person is recovering from cancer treatment. Also, if the purpose of the sessions is to treat a medical condition brought on by the cancer or its treatment, such as when working with lymphedema, adhesions, or scarring, it is prudent to have a written order. I do not ask for written permission if the client has been given a clean bill of health and is seeking massage for relaxation or comfort. Some practitioners may always want to have a written order for their own peace of mind.

Some bodyworkers have wondered if cancer clients should be required to sign a special release of liability form. This is a sticky question. Again, in my opinion, people with cancer should not be singled out and treated any differently than clients without the disease. Asking cancer clients to sign a special release form further stigmatizes them and may plant unnecessary seeds of fear about receiving bodywork. It is incumbent upon the practitioner to learn to give massage in a manner that is safe and creates no risk of liability. If a client requests a technique, pressure, or bodywork to an area that the massage therapist knows is dangerous, the practitioner should explain why she cannot honor the request.

CLIENTS WITH A HISTORY OF CANCER

Lani had been given a gift certificate for a massage from her daughter. She scheduled an appointment during an especially stressful time and was very much looking forward to relaxing. During the intake process Lani indicated a history of skin cancer four years previously. When the massage therapist read this she became unsettled and was uncertain if she should proceed with the session. Lani tried to reassure her that the cure had been complete and that part of her life was over. After more agitated convincing, the practitioner went ahead with the massage, but the tone of fear and doubt had been set and couldn't be overcome.

Responding with apprehension and uncertainty is unnecessary. If a client indicates a history of cancer during intake, the following questions will ascertain what adaptations must be made as well as which modalities could be used to further the client's recovery:

1. When were you diagnosed? What type of cancer was it? Where was it located?

2. What treatment did you receive? When did you finish treatment?

3. Do you see your doctor for check-ups? How often?

4. Do you have any long-term side effects from treatment? Such as:

Sometimes when I go for a massage I don't tell the therapist I am a cancer survivor. They tend to get very nervous, even though I've been cancer free for eight years.

— C.C.

a. neuropathy in the hands or feet
b. osteoporosis
c. fragile veins or easy bruising
d. lymphedema
e. decreased function or range of motion
f. adhesions
g. areas that are sensitive to touch or pressure

Katherine had ovarian cancer eight years ago and had been cancer free during that time, so she thought nothing of it when making an appointment with a new massage therapist. The session, however, never happened. The practitioner refused to work with Katherine without a doctor's note, despite the amount of time that had passed. Bodyworkers who are especially fearful of clients with a history of cancer may want to request written permission for their own peace of mind. However, if the incidence of cancer is several years in the past and a clean bill of health has been given, the session can be approached in exactly the same manner as with a client who has never had cancer. Rather than refusing to massage first time clients until they have doctor's orders, practitioners can work with them using non-invasive techniques such as Reiki or Polarity Therapy. It is very disappointing for clients to be sent away when they have been looking forward to a massage.

TOUCH MODALITIES APPROPRIATE FOR PEOPLE LIVING WITH OR RECOVERING FROM CANCER

Techniques that may be implemented two-three months following the end of treatment and a declaration of remission. Adjustments still may be required with regard to pressure and site restrictions.

Amma	Myotherapy
Aston-Patterning®	Neuromuscular Therapy
Ayurvedic Massage	Russian Massage
Bindegewebsmassage	Seated Chair Massage
Lomilomi (gentle strokes)	Touch for Health
Lymph Drainage Therapies	Trager Psychosocial Integration®
Myofascial Release	Zero Balancing®

Deep bodywork modalities that call for a more lengthy waiting period before administering:

Hellerwork	Postural Integration
Rolfing®	Soma Neuromuscular Integration
Lomilomi (deep strokes)	Thai Massage

These lists are intended only as a general guideline. Each person's unique process must be taken into account when choosing bodywork modalities. The modalities listed on p. 81 are also appropriate for people living with cancer.

Final Thoughts

People with cancer need to be touched. Bodyworkers should be at the forefront in embracing them and in teaching family and friends about the need for touch during this time. Those living with or recovered from cancer should be encouraged to start receiving or continue with bodywork.

Pat had often gone for massage before being diagnosed with cervical cancer, but it didn't occur to her to continue the sessions as she went through surgery and radiation. In retrospect Pat wished that her massage therapist had suggested it. By adapting techniques, reducing the pressure, and avoiding certain sites, the therapist might have been able to assist Pat to find relief from the nausea and fatigue that accompany radiation, and create relaxation, thereby aiding the body's healing process and helping Pat reclaim her body and feel whole again.

A year after treatment Pat returned to massage. By then the meaning of the sessions had changed. Before cancer, the massages had been an extension of her fast-paced life. When the session ended, she immediately stepped back into the high stress, all relaxation quickly forgotten. Now, time spent receiving massage is sacred and meditative. Pat is in the here and now; she tunes into her body; and touch is an experience that helps deepen her awareness. These days, Pat enjoys the good feelings massage brings her body and holds onto those sensations as long as possible. Bodywork helps her let go of the tension, anxiety, and fear that accumulated over the months of treatment.

Massage can be an instrument to help people touch deeper places in themselves.

— G.M.

REFERENCES

1. Frogge, M.H. and M. Goodman. Surgical Therapy in *Cancer Nursing: Principles and Practice*. Boston: Jones and Bartlett, 1987.

2. Chamness, A. Massage Therapy and Persons Living with Cancer. *Massage Therapy Journal*. 1993; 32(3):53-65.

3. Alexander, D. Deep Vein Thrombosis: The Silent Killer. *Nurse's Touch*. 1995; 1(1):16.

4. Romero, R. Massage and Damage to the Lymphatics. *Nurse's Touch*. 1995; 1(1):11.

5 Foldi, E. Editorial: Massage and Damage to Lymphatics. *Lymphology*. 1995; 28:1-3.

6. Hellman, S. and E.E. Vokes. Advancing Current Treatments for Cancer. *Scientific American*. 1996; 275(3):118-123.

7. National Institutes of Health. *Chemotherapy and You*. 1993.

8. Scott, D.; D. Donahue; R. Mastrovito; and T. Hakes. The Antiemetic Effect of Clinical Relaxation: Report of an Exploratory Pilot Study. *Journal of Psychosocial Oncology*. 1983; 1(1):71-83.

9. Skidmore-Roth, L. *Nursing Drug Reference*. St. Louis: Mosby-Year Book, 1998.

10. Shapiro, T.W.; D.B. Davison; and D.M. Rust. *A Clinical Guide to Stem Cell and Bone Marrow Transplantation*. Sudbury, MA: Jones and Bartlett, 1997.

11. Duncan, J.H.; O.M. Colvin; and C. Fenselau. Mass Spectrometric Study of the Distribution of Cyclophosphamide in Humans. *Toxicology and Applied Pharmacology*. 1973; 24:317-323.

12. Madsen, E.S. and H. Larsen. Excretions of Mutagens in Sweat from Humans Treated with Anti-Neoplastic Drugs. *Cancer Letters*. 1988; 40:199-202

13. Foley, K.M. Controlling the Pain of Cancer. *Scientific American*. 1996; 275(3):164-165.

14. Hilderley, L.J. Radiotherapy in *Cancer Nuring: Principles and Practice*. Boston: Jones and Bartlett, 1987

15. National Institutes of Health. *Radiation Therapy and You*. 1990.

16. Piasecki, P.A. Bone Malignancies in *Cancer Nursing: Principles and Practice*. Boston: Jones and Bartlett, 1987.

17. Crawford, J. Myofascial Release Provides Symptomatic Relief From Chest Wall Tenderness Occasionally Seen Following Lumpectomy and Radiation in Breast Cancer Patients. *International Journal of Oncology, Biology, and Physics*. 1996;34(5): 1188-1189.

18. Dunn, T. and M. Williams. *Massage Therapy Guidelines for Hospital and Home Care*. San Francisco: Planetree. 1996.

Chapter 6

BE-ing is Enough:

Comforting Touch for the Dying

In the late 1960's and early '70's, many people re-embraced the idea and practice of giving birth at home. As result, most hospitals now provide a home-like atmosphere that fully incorporates the family into this holy event. At about the same time that home birthing was making a comeback, a similar, but quieter, renaissance was happening as the modern-day hospice movement began. It, once again, placed the care for the dying in the hands of family with help from a team of health care professionals.

Interestingly, these two parts of life, birth and death, have comparable stages. Even so, death is generally not accorded the same sacred status as birth. It is instead regarded as a failure by some, and at the very least as an unwelcome event by most. Many patients and caregivers, however, have found comfort in approaching the end of life just as they would the birth of a long-awaited child. And just as home births are attended by a midwife, so too is home death. These midwives are the caregivers, family, friends, and home health care staff who approach the death of their loved one or patient as a blessed, miraculous event, lovingly prepared for; they commit to be "present throughout [the] journey toward death"[1]; to courageously accompany them to the doorway of the next world.

What does it mean to travel with a person who is dying? It means being able to temporarily leave a world that is earthly, solid, and linear and enter into a state that is ephemeral, porous, and circular. The life of a person who is healthy has a forward-moving pattern to it. The weeks and months of this life can be plotted out more or less on a straight line. On Monday she does this, on Tuesday she does that, and on Wednesday she does something else. The days in the life of an ill or dying person are indistinguishable from one another. Time becomes circular. Sunday is no different from Wednesday. Each day circles into the next, spinning a hazy cocoon around those caught its web. The dying person cannot come "out" to us, we must go "in" to them. We must travel between two worlds, leaving behind the world of do-ing, moving, and productivity to enter a world of be-ing, stillness, and reflection.

Relationships often revolve around what we do together, but when illness and death become part of life, there must be a transition from "doing" to "being." New ways to relate must be found. Massage can bridge the gap between do-ing and be-ing and help us to enter into the world of the person who is at the end of life. Through massage we can simultaneously be "doing" while "being" with our friend, client, or family member.

TOUCH AT THE END OF LIFE

Just as touch is one of the first forms of communication a newborn receives, it may be one of the final ways we talk to the person who is dying. Unfortunately, many caregivers are ill-at-ease about touching someone who is dying, uncertain about what will feel good or fearful of hurting them. As Jan Bernard and Miriam Schneider point out, "When an infant is not nurtured with touch and caring, he does not thrive. When a dying person is not cared for in the same way, she cannot achieve all the healing possible through the process of dying."[1] Through the act of compassionate touch, bodyworkers can be instrumental in showing families that despite the decline in their loved one's body, it is not something to be afraid of. The body of someone who is in the last stage of life, even though frail and dependent, is worthy of the same tenderness, care, and unconditional love as that of a new baby.

In his classic book, *Birth Without Violence*, French obstetrician Fredrich LeBoyer gives us clues about touching the newborn. But they could just as well be instructions for touching the one who is departing:

> *The baby is on the first step of a glorious adventure — and yet it is transfixed with fear. Do not move. Do not add to the baby's*

...touching becomes a way to communicate God's love

— BRADLEY ENERSON

panic. Just be there. Without moving. Without getting impatient. Without asking anything. At this point, out of consideration for her child, out of real – not egocentric – love, a woman will simply place her hands on its body. And leave them there, immobile. Hands that are not animated, agitated, trembling with emotion, but are calm and light. Hands of peace. Through such hands flow the waves of love which will assuage her baby's anguish.[2]

During the last stages of life, there is a place for touch given by a professional massage practitioner and by family and friends. Like an infant, the dying person needs to be touched frequently, not just during the weekly, or even twice weekly, sessions a professional might give. Having a professional's help, however, provides respite for caregivers and gives the patient someone to interact with who is not in the immediate social circle. Patients sometimes withhold information or feelings from their loved ones, believing they are protecting them from further emotional pain. Callanan and Kelley refer to this as a "compassionate conspiracy."[3] During the relaxed atmosphere of a massage session, the one who is dying may feel freer to admit things she has been withholding. The touch practitioner may become a witness to thoughts or feelings the patient still wants to share. Ron, who was dying of leukemia, felt everyone around him was walking on egg shells. No one showed their true feelings or talked to him about his. It was only during his Reiki sessions that he could let down.

Connie, a bone marrow transplant patient who was nearing the end of life in the hospital, also withheld information from her family. Before and after each massage, the massage students at OHSU ask the patients to rate their pain, fatigue, physical and emotional comfort. Connie's husband was in the room while the student collected this information. Initially Connie rated her comfort as fairly high, but as soon as her husband left the room, she changed her ratings, admitting that she was very uncomfortable and in pain.

TEACHING FAMILY TO GIVE MASSAGE

One of the major contributions a bodyworker can make is to instruct family caregivers on basic massage strokes or touch techniques and to encourage them to follow their heart about ways to touch the dying person. When Jane's father was dying of throat cancer, she wished someone had suggested massage to her. Not only did the cancer leave him unable to speak, but he was also deaf, leaving Jane sitting at his bedside feeling helpless and disconnected. By the simple act of stroking his skin, Jane could have communicated with her father, conveying the love she felt through her hands.

Most people have an innate instinct about giving massage, and need only a little tutoring. Touch is the language spoken between mother and child, lover and the beloved, comforter and sufferer. The massage therapist can build on this and teach family and friends other forms of touch and areas of the body that may benefit from

To ease another's heartache is to forget one's own.
— ABRAHAM LINCOLN

Often, touching brings the greatest comfort and is ultimately the healing needed for the heart for both the care giver and care receiver.
— JAN SELLIKEN BERNARD
AND MIRIAM SCHNEIDER,
THE TRUE WORK OF DYING

touch. One of the best ways to teach family and friends is for the practitioner to have the family member work side-by-side with him, each massaging a foot, hand, or leg. The family massage giver can then experience how gentle the touch must be, can emulate the slow, tranquil pace, and can get a better sense of timing.

Health care workers at the VA Medical Center Hospice in Palo Alto have seen the family unit strengthened through massage. They believe it to be a method that assists patients and families to communicate more openly, and has "the effect of strengthening the family bonds in a time of crisis."[4] Helen Campbell, a massage therapist in the Palo Alto program, tells the story of a lung cancer patient who had been estranged for years from his 17 year-old son. The man wished to see his boy before dying. The son reluctantly agreed to come and sit in his father's room, but did not want to talk to his father. When the young man arrived, Helen was massaging his father's feet. The son "sat down noisily in a chair by the window, as far away as possible from his father. His body language was full of resentment." Eventually, however, Helen was able to coax the boy up to where she was and to work alongside of her on his father's other foot. When this raging son put his hands on his father's foot, everything changed. Forgiveness happened "in the giving and receiving of gentle, caring touch."[5] Helen did not have to massage the man again, because the son came every evening after that and massaged him.

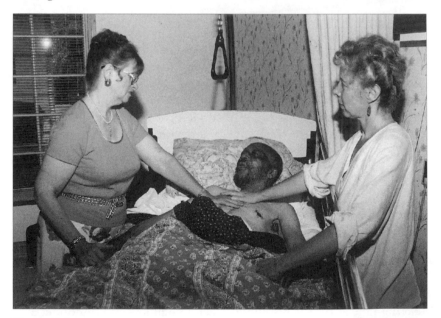

Figure 6-1.

The family massage givers can also learn to use subtle energy techniques by working with the bodyworker. (Figure 6-1.) One night on the way out of the hospital, a student and I were stopped by an excited and grateful family member. Both this student and I had, at different times, worked with this woman's husband who was dying of leukemia. The first time I worked with Bernie, I asked Vivian, his wife, if she would like to give Reiki with me. I thought she would be agreeable because as I worked earlier in the evening with Bernie's roommate, I watched Vivian trying to massage the cramps from her husband's hands. Vivian stood across from me on the other side of the bed and mirrored my hand positions. We spent a peaceful half hour together in silent communion. Bernie fell asleep early on. When he awoke at the end, the cramps, which were unaffected by traditional massage strokes, were gone.

Vivian was stopping us in the hall that night to report that on that particular morning she had been able to use the energy techniques I had taught her all those months ago. Bernie was agitated and in pain. The medications weren't working. So she laid her hands on him as she and I had done. He was soon asleep. But what was so exciting to Vivian was for the first time she was able to "sense" or "see" the source of Bernie's physical pain, which was in his back.

Skilled, supportive touch offers the same benefits for those who are at the end of life as it does for those who are in the middle of life. It helps dying persons know they are important and loved. Hospice nurse Alina Egerman believes that massage allows the person who is dying to escape reality for a moment. "We all need a vacation periodically," says Egerman. "When we can get away for awhile, life often looks different when we return." During massage, the recipient becomes quiet and is able to get in touch with what he is feeling. Gentle massage can help the patient surrender to the process and let go of the body. Ron felt clarity and peace of mind from the touch sessions he received from Reiki Master Sheila King. His acceptance of the situation made it possible for Ron to help his mother let go of him.

Reiki Master Phil Morgan assembled a team of practitioners to provide Reiki for his wife when she was diagnosed with pancreatic cancer. Originally, the team hoped that the disease would be defeated, but eventually they were forced to let go and allow her process to unfold in its own unique way. Phil felt that because of the healing, supportive touch, his wife needed less pain medication which allowed her to be less drugged and more present with her experience. The Reiki helped Phil's wife let go, moving her through to death more quickly and gracefully than anyone had anticipated.

ALLOWING FLEXIBLE BOUNDARIES

Being midwife to a dying friend or loved one is not "business as usual" for the professional bodyworker. Sessions no longer fit neatly into a limited block of time. Instead of an hour, the practitioner/ friend may give touch over a period of hours. When Ron was dying in the hospital, Reiki Master Sheila King administered Reiki for four to five hours at a time. This relieved his discomfort and gave him the opportunity to rest.

The professional massage therapist will be accustomed to following a code of conduct concerning boundaries, both physical

I have often seen...that people who are very sick long to be touched, long to be treated as living people, not diseases. A great consolation can be given to the very ill simply by touching their hands, looking into their eyes, gently massaging them or holding them in your arms, or breathing in the same rhythm gently with them.

— SOGYAL RINPOCHE,
THE TIBETAN BOOK OF THE LIVING AND DYING

and emotional boundaries. However, when caring for a friend or family member who is dying, the boundaries may need to be more flexible to allow for giving care at the deepest level. During Reiki sessions with Ron, Sheila would crawl into bed with him when giving touch to his head. Although a practitioner would not use such a position with a healthy person, lying in bed and holding the person who is at the end of life may be the touch that is needed in that moment.

The emotional boundaries become fuzzy when caring for a person with whom there is a strong attachment; removing the agenda becomes more difficult. The therapist/friend may become impatient, wanting the person who is sick to get well, to be fixed. Although being midwife for someone special is a rewarding experience, it is much more difficult than caring for a person the therapist does not know well. There is no recipe for unfolding these relationships. As best as they can, the midwives must to try to put aside their preconceived notions about how the experience should occur and allow the loved one to direct her own dying.

Some people are averse to receiving massage during this time. They are afraid if they relax too deeply they will let go and die. Touch professionals must honor this position and not push patients to accept massage if they are clearly against it. One of the tenets of hospice care is to allow the patient to control his experience.

SHARING TIME TOGETHER

Anyone who is providing touch for someone at the end of life, whether it be for a client or one's own family member, will want to read some of the books available on this subject. One short chapter is not enough to convey what is known about such topics as communication, grief, or what death will be like. A few basic guidelines for sharing time together are given below:

- **Listening is enough.** Listening is an act complete in itself, but believing that it is enough is difficult. Rachel Naomi Remen speaks often of listening and healing, reminding us that the simple human interaction of listening is the most powerful tool of healing. Healing is accomplished not by doing something, but by receiving the person.[6] People change when they are received and listened to.

  Bodyworkers are natural listeners. They have learned to move into a quiet, still space, to listen with their hands, to hear the non-verbal messages of the body, to communicate without words. In just this same manner they must allow their ears to hear, their voices to respond, to receive the dying one just as they are.

Listening does not require a response. We put ourselves under a strain when we believe a response is necessary and the effort gets in the way of hearing. Listening is effortless. To listen is to be relaxed and quiet. It happens in a silent mind.

— *DARLENE STEWART*

- **Follow the conversational leads of the patient.** Never force the conversation onto topics that the patient does not want to discuss, but if they do initiate the subject of their illness, allow them to talk about it rather than diverting attention away. Many well-meaning visitors try to distract the dying person with talk about what is going on in the outside world, the weather, what's happening at work, or gossip about family and friends. Visitors wrongly suppose that letting the conversation drift toward intimate topics such as death, fear, or the afterlife, will upset their dying friend. More often than not the patient will be grateful for the opportunity to share honest feelings. Despite the attention of many loving people, illness can be a lonely experience when there is no one who understands and accepts the perceptions of the ill person.

- **Smile and laugh.** Serious illness does not put a ban on laughter.

- **Allow silence.** Love needs no words and silence can be as supportive and welcome as conversation. As death approaches, the one who is dying will withdraw and words become less important. The giving and receiving of touch allows both people to spend quiet time together in a pleasurable, undemanding way that needs no words.

- **You don't have to have all the answers.** In the PBS documentary, When Doctors Get Cancer, Dr. Balfour Mount says, "As caregivers we think we have to have the answers. [But] we don't have the answers. If we are there to share the questions, that's what the person wants [and] needs."[7] At times there are no complete solutions. Accept that you are limited and do what you are able to.

- **Don't offer untrue statements.** If a patient isn't doing well, don't make remarks such as: "You'll be good as new before you know it." Or, "You're probably feeling down because of the weather." Acknowledge their feelings and the situation as it actually is with comments such as, "It sounds as if you're really uncomfortable", or "You seem frustrated."

- **Respect the privacy, wishes, and beliefs of the patient.** Call before you visit. Never assume you know what is best for them. Don't force your ides about illness or death onto the patient. Allow him to have his experience as he would like.

- **Be there to support the person's process.** Have no agenda or expectations. Massage professionals are sometimes at a loss when they make a visit expecting to give a massage, only to have the patient decline. It is best to have no expectations about how the time will be spent. The focus should be on spending time together not on massage.

The basic quality that makes people helpful to other sentient beings is compassion.

— THE DALAI LAMA,
LIVING AND DYING IN JOY AND PEACE

- **Offer to help, but only if you can follow through.** Don't make idle offers. In their book *Final Gifts*, Maggie Callanan and Patricia Kelley suggest offering to help with specific tasks.[3] Rather than making a general comment such as, "Let me know how I can help", ask the patient (or caregiver) if you could do the grocery shopping once a week, take the kids to soccer practice, mow the lawn, or massage her feet. People who are in the final stages of life usually do not have the energy or even the interest to compile "to-do" lists when friends casually ask if there is some way they can help.

- **Allow the person to do what she can for herself.** Most people want to be as independent as possible for as long as possible.

- **Give the one who is ill the opportunity to not only be a receiver of help but also a giver of help.** Everyone wants to feel useful. Caregivers need to permit themselves to be receivers whenever possible. Not only will the dying one feel they are making a contribution, but caregivers will feel less burnout.

SUPPORTING LIFE UNTIL THE END

You matter until the last moment of your life, and we will do all we can not only to help you die peacefully but also to live until you die.

— DR. CICELY SAUNDERS,
FOUNDER OF THE MODERN-DAY
HOSPICE MOVEMENT
AND OF ST. CHRISTOPHER'S HOSPICE
IN ENGLAND

When the physician feels that the patient has six months or less to live, the person can choose to enroll in a hospice program. The goal of hospice care is no longer to search for a cure, but to manage symptoms palliatively, allowing the patient's remaining time to be as peaceful and comfortable as possible. The hospice staff of doctors, nurses, social workers, physical and occupational therapists, massage therapists, and chaplains works with the family to care for the patient at home or in a home-like setting. Although not all cancer patients choose to die at home or to be served by a hospice agency, the hospice philosophy can be implemented anywhere. Hospice is not a place, it is a "concept of care"[3] that emphasizes helping patients live fully until the end.

People's dying process is as unique as their births or their lives, for that matter. Some patients remain fairly active until the last month and then quickly slip away. Others slowly decline over several years. The person with cancer who is preparing to depart this world will follow a series of stages that more or less are the reverse of those in the birthing process. These stages are especially applicable to the cancer process which unfolds slowly, unlike the suddenness of death caused by a heart attack. Familiarity with the stages of dying may help the bodyworker understand the behavior she observes from her dying friend or family member, and therefore be more present with the process. Because the experience of giving birth is well-known to many, it will be used as a springboard to understanding the stages of dying. The timelines, however, may not always follow those given in the sections below.

QUICKENING — A Few Months Prior to Death

Around the fifth month, the fetus usually makes its presence known by kicking, stretching, and shifting within the womb. These first movements, referred to as the "quickening,"[8] are a time of excitement for the expecting parents, friends, and family. Placing a hand on the mother's swelling abdomen to feel these signs of life is a moment full of awe, curiosity, and excitement.

Death, too, often makes its presence known by some defining movement. These movements are not as noticeable, dramatic, or welcomed as those delivered by the developing fetus, and they may only be evident in hindsight. Ralph threw a big party for his friends the Christmas before he died, but may not have been conscious that death was becoming present when he did so. However, when his friends looked back, they could see that it was his way of saying good-bye. Six or seven months before his death, Charles and his ex-wife prepared an advanced medical directive to insure that no heroic

ROGER

Roger, a 41 year-old man with brain cancer, requested I come to his home and massage him on a regular basis. His doctor had OK'd via a written script. I struggled with the strong influence from my schooling that said "massage was contraindicated for cancer patients", but I accepted the contract because my intuitive feeling was that massage would help Roger manage pain, stress, and nausea, and provide self-esteem and nurturing. The patient had been receiving chemotherapy, but these treatments were stopped around the time the massage sessions began.

Roger's home was busy with his young children, visitors, business and financial matters, and lots of tension. Avoiding interruptions was impossible. The sessions generally consisted of Swedish Massage, range of motion (ROM) exercises, and Myofascial Release techniques. His arms were asymmetrical in size and strength, similar to a stroke, with weakness and frozen joints in the arms and legs on the effected side. Early on we also did some muscle strengthening to help him propel the wheelchair. Gradually this type of session gave way to quieter, slower effleurage, holding and stroking, with gentle, careful ROM. The stretching became too painful.

At first I think Roger was desperate for anything that might reverse the cancer, or get it into remission. He would ask about herbal and alfalfa additives. I explained that short of a miracle, massage could not undo the process, but could add to his comfort. He wanted to continue. I wanted the miracle.

Near the end, keeping Roger at home was too difficult and he was moved to a skilled care facility. I visited him there, not purposely to give massage, but I always laid a hand on him, stroked his forehead, or massaged hands and feet. He had stopped talking, and his head listed to one side. For awhile he could squeeze a hand in response. His eyes took on a fixed stare, no facial expression. It was difficult to know what he wanted to convey. Death came shortly after.

There was a spiritual element running through this period of dying, but that is another whole story — private and exhilarating for me to witness. I believe I got my miracle, of sorts, though not a physical healing. I felt privileged to give Roger massage during the final few months of his life. I learned how to adjust the techniques, depth of massage, and positioning to the patient's changing condition. Roger's wife and mother expressed their gratitude for the way it helped him. An additional benefit for me was the chance to follow my intuition and the rationale of the heart, opting for the greater good, one of nurturing, comforting human touch at a time of great need.

— J.A., R.N., L.M.T.

*Where is my patient, Mrs. D? At
times she appears to converse with
me; in other moments she seems
worlds away. Is this due to her
medication, fatigue, or brain
metastases:*

Maybe she's in her garden.

*As I gently massage her arms and
draw down to and linger on her palms
and fingertips, I can almost feel the
freshened spring soil as she prepares it
for seed. I can feel the calm blossom
in my heart. She loves to make things
grow...*

— J.P., L.M.T.

measures would be taken to keep him alive. Perhaps it was
preparedness that motivated Charles, or perhaps he was becoming
aware of death's proximity. Elsie called a meeting of her five daughters
a few months before her death. One evening they all gathered at the
nursing home where their mother was being cared for to select a piece
of jewelry from Elsie's treasure box.

Whereas the fetus becomes noticeably active during the
"quickening" stage, the person preparing to depart the world becomes
less active. They may sleep and nap more, have less interest in the
outside world, and eat fewer solid foods. The physical life is gradually
left behind.[9] Massage, however, is one physical experience that still
holds pleasure.

MASSAGE COMFORT MEASURES

- During the quickening stage, bodywork sessions will be
  similar to those for people in treatment or for hospitalized
  patients. By and large, light to moderate pressure is used,
  with the emphasis on relaxation. The patient may need
  more assistance, may have position restrictions due to
  tumors or medical devices, sessions may need to be shorter
  or may need to be conducted in the home. John was
  housebound for several months prior to his death, but
  continued receiving massage at home until the end. He
  insisted on receiving the sessions on a portable massage
  table rather than in his bed because he wanted to feel
  normal for as long as possible. Another homebound client
  also wanted to receive her sessions on a massage table. The
  therapist was able to help the patient accomplish this by
  raising the hospital bed to the same height as the massage
  table and then helping the patient roll onto the table.
  Esther, on the other hand, was still able to drive herself to
  weekly Reiki sessions and climb 13 stairs to the treatment
  room during this stage.

- People with cancer, especially in the end stage of life, may
  be on morphine and codeine preparations to manage their
  pain. One of the side effects of narcotics is the slowing
  down of the bowel which creates constipation. Kik
  Lovegren instructs her hospice clients or caregivers how to
  do two minutes of clockwise abdominal massage in the
  morning and evening to assist the bowels.

- Fatigue may increase due to anemia from radiation or bone
  marrow changes. Lack of nutrition caused by nausea or the
  inability to absorb nutrients may also contribute to
  tiredness. Fatigue can result in the patient doing less for
  herself, becoming inactive, or communicating less.
  Anecdotal evidence suggests that massage is effective in
  temporarily reducing fatigue for some people, especially a
  full-body session, whether Swedish Massage or a subtle
  energy technique is used.

- Administering massage to the joints and performing passive or active range of motion exercises can contribute to patients' overall comfort, allow them to do more for themselves, and make it easier for care partners to provide care. The more mobile the patient is, the easier it is to accomplish daily care activities such as dressing, going to the bathroom, or turning in bed.

LIGHTENING —
A Few Days to a Few Weeks Prior to Death

A few days to a few weeks before delivery, the fetus begins to move into the delivery position, usually with the head turned down toward the birth canal. In obstetrics this stage is referred to as "lightening."[8] This is the beginning of moving from an internal reality to an external one. During this time the baby takes in a lot of nutrition and puts on weight.

Conversely, a few days to a few weeks before entering the active phase of dying, the person will prepare by withdrawing from the outside world and move inward. (Figure 6-2.) Eating and drinking decrease, weight is lost, and breathing patterns and rates may vary. The patient's breathing may speed up one moment, slow down in the next, or may stop altogether for a short period of time before returning to an even pace.[1] These changes in the breath are due to

(continued on page 114)

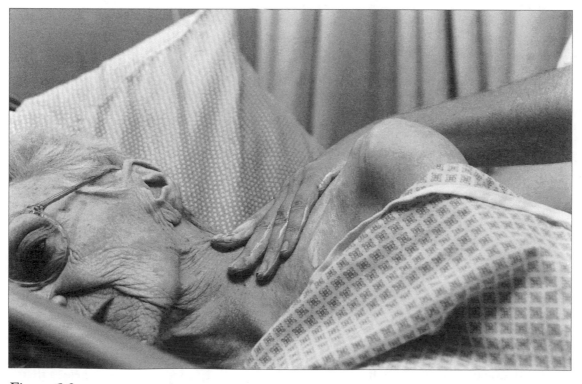

Figure 6-2.

PAUL

I am an RN who has experience with dying patients, but Paul was the first close friend to have a terminal illness. He was diagnosed with colon cancer 18 months before. The onset was sudden and shocking to his two sons and wife. He endured chemotherapy, which he had thought he would not survive. The next Christmas the cancer had metastasized to his stomach and other parts of the colon. As part of an experimental procedure he was going to have abdominal surgery to remove the tumors. This was to be followed by a heated chemotherapy treatment. However, when they opened him up the cancer was everywhere, so they closed him up and sent him home with four months to live.

My husband, children, and I flew to visit Paul, knowing that it would be to say good-bye. It had been six years since we had seen each other. These were not the most favorable conditions for a reunion. Last time we were together, I was working as an OB nurse. This time, I was studying to be a massage therapist.

It was awkward and difficult to see a 44 year-old man who we remembered as very fit and full of life look so frail and weak. His skin was waxy and pale. Tumors were obstructing his bowel and causing pressure on the abdomen making it impossible for him to eat. Paul looked like a prisoner of war. Slowly he was starving to death, uncertain which would kill him first, the cancer or the starvation. He had an IV in his left arm through which he received fluids 13 hours a day for hydration. Morphine was also being given through the IV via a PCA pump with the dosage being increased more and more frequently.

When we first arrived, we all exchanged stories, catching up on the last six years. The conversation stayed to the pleasantries. There was feeling of unease and not knowing what to say. Eventually the talk came around to massage and Paul related a story about going to a resort for a mud wrap and massage a few months previously when he was stronger. It was so relaxing lying there all wrapped up with warm mud. When they hosed off the mud the water was warm and felt so good.

As he told of his experience, Paul's eyes closed. I could tell it was a very pleasant memory. I asked how his comfort level was now. He answered that he was having a lot of abdominal cramping, pain, was tired all the time, and his body ached from being in bed so much. Certain odors nauseated him and seven or eight times a day he would vomit. I asked if he thought a foot massage might help ease the discomfort. Paul brightened up and emphatically said, "YES".

When I laid my hands on him I felt his fear and restlessness. At first he was very quiet, eyes closed, a smile on his face. When I finished his feet, my friend asked if I would massage his back. I could feel his body relax under my hands. His wife, Sandy, watched with great relief to see her husband feeling truly comfortable.

As I massaged, a bond was being forged. There was a certain unspoken trust between us. Paul knew I was not afraid of him or his illness, that he was not alone. If love can flow through hands, it did. He talked about his fear of dying and leaving his family; about the burden he was now to his wife and boys; and his inability to even be man enough to provide for his family or protect them. I was present. I listened. I continued to massage his back, then moved to the face and head. I had no profound answers or responses to make it all better. God, how I wish I did, though. Paul just wanted someone to listen and hear him; to really care about what he was feeling and was going through. This I could do. I must say, though, that it is much easier to be able to "do" something than it is to just be present, especially when there is a strong emotional tie to the one who is dying.

Paul had fallen asleep. When I finished, I let him sleep. That night he slept nearly the entire night, a rare occurrence. Usually he would wake every few hours and poor Sandy was exhausted. She was so pleased that he finally got some good rest.

The next morning Paul asked if I would massage him again. He derived so much joy from the massage that I was eager to do it. It was a gift to me. Nothing, he told me, brought him joy or pleasure any more except music and the massages. I massaged his back and feet again while he listened to his favorite CD's. Massaging the shoulders was difficult. Paul was so emaciated I was afraid he was going to break. Once again he talked about his sons and how much he was going to miss seeing them grow up. Despite the sadness, my gentle-spirited friend looked better that morning than he had the day before. Even Sandy commented on it. He seemed to have more energy and even wanted to get into the pool with the kids. So, into the water we all went and reminisced about old times.

The remainder of the day went the same. I would give him a massage, he would fall asleep, waking up rejuvenated. It almost gave us hope that he was getting better, but it was only false hope.

The night before we left I asked Sandy if she would like a massage. She looked so tired from giving round the clock care without help, except from their 13 and 15 year-old sons. It was the first time in months she had done something for herself. Lying on the massage table gave her time to think and reflect, to regroup for a few hours. We discussed Paul's memorial service and picked out pictures, talked about the cremation and where to spread the ashes, and spoke of finances and how to keep the house and send the boys to college. I don't think we left a stone unturned in the conversation. Having someone else to acknowledge that she was going to lose her husband of 17 years and would be left to raise two sons alone relieved her sense of isolation. Several times the conversation brought up tears, but we were also able to laugh. Both Paul and Sandy commented that they hadn't realized how little laughter there was in the house now. Having friends around to share old memories brought a laughter that showered us all with feelings of safety and belonging. It was a healthy grieving process for us all. They did not try to hide anything from the boys or each other. Everything was talked about openly, including Paul's death and what it might be like.

I learned so much from those few days. It was very difficult, but the massage eased the way and was truly a healing act for us all. The touch became a way to communicate without trying to figure out what to say and how to say it. Teaching families a few basic massage strokes would not only help the patient, but would give caregivers and friends a way to bridge that initial awkwardness. I watched as Paul's visitors clumsily tried to avoid the big elephant in the room. Everyone saw it, but nobody would talk about it. In their helplessness they would either talk non-stop about everything and nothing or would lapse into uncomfortable silence. If these people just knew how to rub Paul's back or feet, it would have opened the lines of communication. One thing Paul did when he received massage was talk.

Our final good-byes were the hardest I've ever had to say. My heart was pounding and the words were choked. This experience has changed me forever. I am closer to God and truly value and appreciate my family and my life. Life is a gift that should not be left unopened.

Two weeks after we left, Paul died. What he gave me was so valuable that a part of him will stay with me always. As an OB nurse I always felt honored to be present at births. Helping to bring a new life into the world was a joyous celebration. There is an aura about birth that makes you want to bask in it. Now I know after being with my friend that I want to help the terminally ill in their final months to make the transition from life to death with caring, grace, comfort, and love.

— C.F.

R.N., L.M.T.

the decrease in circulation causing body wastes to build-up.[10] Other changes may be:

Skin: Fragile; pressure sores; rashes; bruising; bleeding; skin color may fluctuate from flushed to bluish or a pale yellow (not to be confused with the yellow of jaundice); the hands, feet, and nailbeds may become pale and bluish as the circulation slows.

GI Tract: Nausea; vomiting; constipation or diarrhea; dry or sore mouth.

Musculoskeletal: Weakness; fatigue; loss of movement; brittle bones.

Emotional: Can range from calm and accepting to anxious and agitated; depression; anger; impatience; restless; picking at the bed covers and other agitated arm movements. Some hospice workers believe these random appearing arm motions are actually an indication that the dying person is experiencing something and that the picking and agitated arm movements are an attempt to communicate with someone who can only be seen by them.[3]

General: Pain may be present for some and absent for others; body temperature may fluctuate; varied sleeping and waking patterns; sensitivity to sights, smells, sounds, and movement; incontinent.

MASSAGE COMFORT MEASURES

- If the patient is able to communicate, ask them directly, rather than the family or caregivers, what they want from the massage session.[10]

- When offering to give massage, especially to someone who has not had one since becoming ill, make the offer specific, such as "Would you like your feet gently massaged?" Most people do not realize that massage can just be given to a part of the body or that the pressure can be adapted to meet the needs of someone who is dying. They often imagine it will be a vigorous rub-down of the entire body rather than a soft, comforting experience.

- The range of bodywork given during this time is still fairly broad. Some people may want a light, full-body massage, others may want only parts of the body massaged, (Figure 6-3) or just to have their hand held.

- Create privacy for the massage recipient if possible and appropriate. The dying one often will be surrounded by family and friends during this time. Ask the patient if he would prefer to have family remain in the room or would rather receive massage in private. Many people are more able to fully relax when they are left to themselves. In addition, the massage session is an opportune time for family and friends to refresh themselves with a walk, nap, or meal.

- Use increased gentleness when touching people at this stage. The skin and flesh may be tender or bones may be brittle.

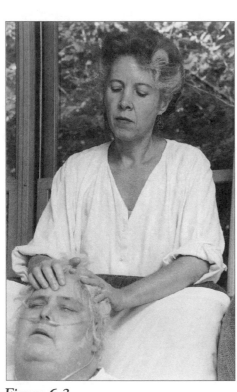

Figure 6-3

- Skin care is vital for people confined to bed. If they can tolerate it, patients should be massaged daily with lotion. This will increase circulation and moisturize the skin, decreasing the chance of pressure sores developing. Maintaining skin integrity becomes even more important as people lose weight. Pressure occurs where bones are close to the surface causing the skin to break down and possibly allowing the bone to break through.[11] Massage the skin covering joints to maintain its suppleness in these high risk areas.

- If a patient has a stage 1 pressure sore (reddened but intact skin), do not directly massage the spot as further damage may be caused, especially in older cancer patients whose skin has less elasticity and integrity. When massaging in the vicinity of a pressure sore, leave a one inch buffer of healthy skin.

- Incorporate other activities into the massage time, such as music, aromatherapy, or relaxation imagery. Some people enjoy having guided meditations, prayers, or stories read to them. In his books *Healing into Life and Death* and *Guided Meditations, Explorations and Healings*, Stephen Levine has many wonderful meditations on pain, taking medications, letting go, and dying.

- Say good-bye each time when working with someone who has entered this phase of dying; leave nothing undone or unsaid with a person when you leave.[10]

As the patient enters the final few weeks of life, eating and drinking decrease. Because food and drink are equated with nurturing, caregivers are often at a loss about how to provide sustenance.[12] Loving, gentle touch can be a form of nourishment, a spiritual nourishment that feeds caregivers and care receivers.

ACTIVE LABOR —
A Few Hours to a Few Days Prior to Death

Active labor, or the onset of regular contractions, is the sign that the birthing process has begun. These contractions progressively create the opening in preparation for delivery of the baby. This process can begin hours or sometimes days before the actual birth. The one who is dying undergoes a comparable process a few hours to a few days before death. Active labor for the dying person is a series of physical processes that progressively shut down the body. The changes that occurred during the "lightening" phase generally become more intense. Additional changes that may occur are:

Skin: Extremities cool to the touch; mottling; lips and nails turn blue, hands and feet turn purplish; backside of the body becomes blotchy as well as the ankles, knees, and elbows.

Hands that know the art of touch as "anointing", and treat the body as "sacrament" will never be without work... Massage as the art of anointing is a vocation, a call to loving work through our hands... If our hands are prayers, then touching another person as in massage... is indeed an embodied way of praying our care for another person.

— MARY ANN FINCH,
FOUNDER AND DIRECTOR OF THE
CENTER FOR GROWTH IN WHOLENESS

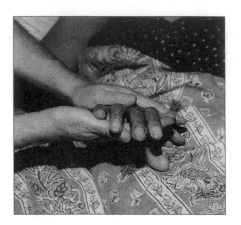

Figure 6-4.

GI Tract: Difficulty swallowing.

Breathing: Breathing pattern becomes very irregular; mucous gathers in mouth and congests in the throat or lungs causing the loud breathing sound known as the "death rattle;" there may be loud moans or sighs as the "letting go of life occurs."[1]

Musculoskeletal: Weak and unable to do anything for self; unable to turn in bed; twitches; restless.

Mental Functions: Decreased awareness; inability to concentrate; can still hear even if other senses have faded.

Emotional: May be calm and accepting or fearful and anxious; may relax when family members are at the bedside.[1]

Spiritual: Out-of-body events; sense of connection to spiritual source;[1] may have a sudden surge of energy in which they are able to clearly speak to those around them or may wish to share a meal despite not wanting food for the preceding weeks.[3]

General: Sleep deepens, making the patient more difficult to rouse; deterioration of body causing odors, incontinence, and secretions; urine output decreases and urine darkens.

MASSAGE COMFORT MEASURES:

Continue touch to the end unless the person cannot tolerate or is distracted by it. It may be as simple as holding his hand or lying in bed and cradling her. (Figure 6-4.)

MRS. YEANG

Mrs. Yeang, diagnosed with terminal gall bladder cancer, was admitted to hospice in order to receive quality care at home in her final days. In the short time I spent with the Yeangs, I watched love and strength grow amid fear and pain, saw Mrs. Yeang's growing comprehension of her transition, and her husband's strength in the face of confusion, helplessness, and loss. I saw the youngest daughter's optimism and logic juxtaposed with her older, pregnant sister's vacillation between sorrow for her dying mother and excitement about the upcoming birth of her child. This experience with the Yeangs helped prepare me in a great degree for my mother's death, which followed just four and a half weeks later.

I'll never forget my final session at the Yeangs. Upon entering the house I was greeted by Michelle, the youngest daughter. A warm silence, punctuated with subdued voices and the rattle of utensils, came from the kitchen. I was given a cup of green tea. Lunch was over and most of the family was there. Though Mrs. Yeang's health had declined since I had last seen her, there was a sense of quietude about her that balanced out the failing of her body. Despite chapped lips, a dry blistered mouth, and a frail, failing body, she lay ready to receive massage.

I sat down and laid my hand within Mrs. Yeang's. I manipulated her left palm and metacarpals, working my way out to each finger. She lay there in appreciation and acceptance. A transparent light seemed to emanate from her and reflect to the snowflakes drifting outside the living room windows. It was odd being enthralled by the beauty of Mrs. Yeang and the snow-covered evergreens and boulders.

Mrs. Yeang's fingers seemed longer that day, her arms a bit thinner. Seeking out the proper pressure and glide on her drying skin showed me just how much in my head I was. How do I keep my heart open and still be effective technically? How do I touch someone whose body is drifting away? How can I properly sit within this moment? Who is really touching whom? Mrs. Yeang was teaching but I didn't know I was her student. Now, more than a year later,

- Many hospice workers have commented that touching the body during the final days and hours seems to distract the dying person from letting go, bringing the attention back to the body. If this seems to be happening, hold and touch her energetically in your mind and heart as you sit with her. Even if you never put your hands on the one who is departing, it doesn't mean you haven't touched him. What is most needed at the end is presence, not doing.

- If the dying one cannot be touched directly, smooth the energy field above him with a long, effleurage type of stroke.

- Ascertaining tolerance for touch when the dying one is unresponsive can be difficult. Some practitioners prefer not to give touch to these patients in case it causes pain which the patient is unable to communicate. Subtle cues such as eye movements or breathing rate may indicate discomfort. However, if the massage giver is concerned about hurting the person who is dying, she can employ the suggestions given in the above sections rather than directly touching the patient.

- Hearing remains acute until death. Even if the person is in a coma, explain who you are and why you are there. For instance, before touching her you might say, "In a minute I am going to put my hands on your feet." From time to time explain what you are doing.[10] Sheila King talks to the

Repeatedly, I am awed that the most wondrous of all the massage strokes is that of simply 'resting' — resting my hands, resting my intentions, resting my heart as one would rest in contemplative prayer. Compassionate massage, then, also embodies contemplation. Silently, I am here, sheltering you through my hands with my own vulnerable and wounded loveliness.

— MARY ANN FINCH

I am beginning to learn from my time with her. I still find it difficult to maintain the higher quality of "the work", to possess active intent and passive mind.

By the time I worked my way to her feet, the snow had started accumulating. Soothing her arches and spreading her metatarsals I watched her daughters console each other with the kindness of touch and food. Yuka, fatigued by grief and pregnancy, sat with eyes closed, warming her hands on a cup of tea. Michelle, having brought dessert for her sister, quietly sat beside her. She watched as I gently soothed and lengthened her mother's calf muscles. Mr. Yeang came to the doorway, carrying anguish, love, and tortured acceptance. I didn't understand his suffering until I saw my father carry the same burden soon after. Even now, I don't totally comprehend their turmoil. I only have hints of it. I haven't spent thirty, forty, or fifty years sharing my life with someone I love, creating a world together, and then slowly losing it. These sufferings are carried as burdens and as blessings. Compassion and the understanding of who we are/were/can be seems to truly blossom only after experiencing love and the hurt of its loss.

I moved to her head to close with some energy work. What I was doing for Mrs. Yeang was good, but it was a crude reflection of the energy work the family was already doing as they sat being present with each other, their love and her love. I would learn more about this in the months that followed. It is important to have the structure of "healing work" and it is important to do the practice of healing and massage, but as the old Zen master said, "Don't mistake the finger for the moon." The real work is being in the process, being a reflection of these healings.

The snow was getting deeper and the forecast was ominous. We decided at the end of Mrs. Yeang's session that I would go home without massaging Michelle and Yuka. After I got my things together, Mrs. Yeang wanted to kiss me good-bye. I brought my forehead to her lips and received her kiss. Thank you, Mrs. Yeang. Later that night she died surrounded by her family.

— Glenn Ben-Ezra, L.M.T.

May the work of your hands be a sign of gratitude and reverence to the human condition.

— MAHATMA GANDHI

dying person with her mind. As she worked with Ron during the last days of his life, he would mentally tell her where to put her hands.

- We touch the dying person not only with our hands, but our eyes, our tone of voice, and even our thoughts.[10] People near death are sensitive to and perceptive of the thoughts and emotions around them.[1] Some hospice workers believe that the unconscious thoughts brought into the room by friends or caregivers can help the situation or can agitate the patient and slow down the dying process. Strive to face the fears or discomforts that arise from being part of someone's dying process. Being honest with yourself about how you feel will make your emotional energy field more calm and clear. If your distress makes it impossible to work in that moment, permit yourself to leave the room. Massage givers must honor their process, too.

Therese Schroeder-Sheker, founder of the Chalice Repose Project, tends to the dying with music specially designed for their needs. She teaches her interns that they must "differentiate between music for the living and music for the dying. Music for the living is meant to" be engaging, whereas music for the dying is meant to be freeing, to help them let go.[13]

Touch for the dying should also be freeing, allowing them to be unfettered rather than binding them to this plane. How could we touch someone in a way that does not hold them back, that allows freedom, and even encourages them to go deeper into the passageway? Our hands and heart must be open, not clutching; they must be light, still, and calm, asking nothing, offering thanks and release. We must create an emotional spaciousness within ourselves that allows the dying person the freedom to be on any plane necessary; and try not to pull the person out of the internal world she has entered and into our external one. The books, *Coma: A Healing Journey* by Amy Mindell and *Final Gifts* by Maggie Callanan and Patricia Kelley, may teach the bodyworker to assist dying people in following their experience.

THE MOMENT OF DEATH

Some births happen with just a few easy pushes while others are a long, drawn out, Herculean task. The moment of death, too, is unique and can happen with gentle ease or struggle and effort. Each death is what it is. Like birth, death is a passage, not a success or failure. It deserves the same honor we reserve for the moment of birth whether it was a peaceful experience or a conflicted one.

At the moment of death, the following changes may occur:

- No pulse
- Skin color changes to gray
- Eyes lose focus and remain open at death

- Breathing gradually stops. It is sometimes difficult to decide if the breathing actually has stopped. The last few breaths may sound like a sigh.[3] Others have described the final breaths as "fish out of water" breathing.[9]

- Involuntary loss of stool or urine[1]

MASSAGE COMFORT MEASURES:

- Continue to move slowly and gently around the body, allowing a sacred space for the transition of spirit.[1] According to many traditions, the soul leaves the body gradually.[12]

- Clean and prepare the body. (See "Judy's Last Massage")

- Say good-bye through prayer, ritual, silent meditation. The good-bye is not only to the one who has died, but also to what has been lost because of the death. For the ones left behind, it often feels as if part of themselves has died. Reading special prayers or spiritual passages may also help the "newly released soul become free of suffering and find its way in the afterlife."[12]

JUDY'S LAST MASSAGE

For years I have received professional massage on a regular basis. When my sister Judy was being treated for a rare form of sarcoma, I thought massage would help her discomfort and tried to convince her to go for a session given by someone trained in the field. Judy, however, wanted me to do it. After being on the receiving end of so many wonderful massages, I needed no instruction, my hands instinctively knew what to do. Judy and I had been competitive swimmers as girls. The long, gliding strokes of massage reminded us of that time, a time that had been especially important to Judy.

I was born prematurely, weighing just under four pounds. When our parents brought me home from the hospital, Judy, who was three years old at the time, heaped love and attention on me. But as we grew up and our personalities evolved, the relationship became somewhat contentious. This continued on into adulthood and was not resolved until Judy's illness. The massage was one of the few ways Judy got relief from pain, but the sessions also played an important role in healing our relationship.

My mother and I were with Judy when she died. After she finally passed, I called the hospice nurse to have them come and take out the tubes, catheter, and remove the PCA pump. After the nurse had disposed of the impersonal, medical side of the experience, I took a new bar of Judy's favorite lavender soap, a wash cloth, and basin of water, and proceeded to clean, clear, rest, and settle her exhausted and spent body. In a rather horrified way, my mother asked what I was doing. I told her I was preparing Judy, not unlike she had done when she brought Judy into this world. My 79 year-old mother became very quiet and thoughtful, but without another word she got a wash cloth and towel and lovingly began to wash Judy's left side while I washed the right. After bathing her frail body, I gently massaged Judy with oil one last time, using the long, flowing strokes that she loved. When the massage ended, we smudged the room with sage and had a quiet time with Judy before calling the mortician. Then my mother and I dressed Judy in her favorite swim suit, a red and orange Hawaiian print that reminded her of swimming in the ocean. Now she was ready for the next big event.

— Mary Blake

Usually, the bodyworker will not be with the patient when death occurs unless she is part of the immediate family. The moment of death, like the moment of birth or sex, is so private that even though a massage therapist may have developed a close, intimate relationship over the months of massaging the patient, the dying person generally wants only a few special people with him at the end. Some people even prefer to have no one with them and will time the moment of death until after everyone has left the room.

During final labor, the patient sometimes feels free to die when she knows that her loved ones are being taken care of. This is something the touch therapist can do. By caring for family members he is indirectly giving help to the dying one.

FINAL THOUGHTS

In 1994, voters in my home state, Oregon, ratified the "Death with Dignity Act", allowing patients who meet certain qualifications to request a prescription from their doctor for a lethal dose of drugs. Although Oregon's laws were enlightened regarding the use of narcotics for pain management and it had a much higher rate of hospice use than the national average, it obviously was not enough to give people a sense of security about the care they would receive at the end of life. This historic legislation was tied up in the courts for years. However, as I wrote this chapter, implementation of the law was allowed for the first time in the cases of four terminal patients.

Also, as I am finishing this chapter, a bodyworker who specializes in giving touch to the dying recounted a discussion she had with a hospice nurse that ended with the nurse stating that "massage is a luxury." If we as a society believed that "massage is a necessity" at every stage of life, and that everyone is valuable, even in dying, how would care for the dying be influenced? And, how would this impact the discussion on physician-assisted suicide?

Eventually, as other communities move to pass similar legislation, this topic will be debated all over the United States and the world. In Oregon, the proposed ballot measure was beneficial in that it brought the conversation about dying and death out into the open. It also issued a wake-up call to the medical establishment. One of the immediate side effects was an examination of the treatment provided to people who are dying. A shift is now underway in Oregon to improve the care for terminally ill people which will make it possible for them to live as comfortably as possible until death, with greater dignity and worth. Since the focus is now on care measures such as pain management, comfort food, music, and spiritual counseling, comfort-oriented touch hopefully will be recognized as a necessary and integral part of care for the dying. Touch practitioners must contribute their ideas about ministering to the dying as the greater conversation unfolds.

The act of giving touch to people at the end of life is simple. Professional bodyworkers may be skilled in a variety of massage modalities, but for people in the last months of life, touch techniques are less important than the quality of the practitioner's presence. Most of us, however, are no longer accustomed to interacting and being present with someone who is dying and must seek out additional training and other sources of information. *Medicine Hands* is only a beginning.

Walking the final steps with someone who is leaving this world is a privilege. The journey can be a meaningful process for the one who is dying and those around her, and is as important as any part of life.[14] I have seen mid-wives to the dying shortly after being present at the death of their friend, patient, or family member. Their countenance is one of awe, light emanates from their face, and they temporarily seem to be on a higher plane. Those who attend a birth often reflect the same brilliance, mystery, and other-worldliness. Like birth, death is holy and worthy of embracing. Loving touch shifts us into that sacred place and reminds us that death is a blessed and miraculous event.

REFERENCES

1. Bernard, J. S. and M. Schneider. *The True Work of Dying: A Practical and Compassionate Guide to Easing the Dying Process.* New York: Avon Books, 1996.

2. LeBoyer, F. *Birth Without Violence.* New York: Knopf, 1975.

3. M. Callanan and P. Kelley. *Final Gifts.* New York: Bantam Books, 1992.

4. Ellis V.; J. Hill; and H. Campbell. Strengthening the Family Unit Through the Healing Power of Massage. *The American Journal of Hospice and Palliative Care.* 1995;12(5):19-21.

5. Campbell, H. Why We Do What We Do: A True Story of Love and Forgiveness. *Hospital Based Massage Newsletter.* 1996;2(3):8-9.

6. Rachel Naomi Remen, interview by Bill Moyers, *Healing and The Mind* video (Wounded Healers segment), 1993.

7. Balfour Mount, interview, *When Doctors Get Cancer,* PBS video: Station WHYY, Philadelphia, 1994.

8. Thomas, C.L., ed. *Taber's Cyclopedic Medical Dictionary.* Philadelphia: F.A. David Co., 1993.

9. Karnes, B. *Gone From My Sight: The Dying Experience.* Self-published, 1986.

10. Nelson, D. *Compassionate Touch: Hands-On Caregiving for the Elderly, the Ill and the Dying.* Barrytown, New York: Station Hill Press, 1994.

11. Huntington, L. *Living with Hope, Dying with Dignity: Home Care for the Terminal Patient.* Master Books Publishers, 1988.

12. Peay, P. *A Good Death.* Common Boundary. 1997;15(5):32-41.

13. Schroeder-Sheker, T. Music for the Dying. *Noetic Sciences Review.* 1994. Autumn. p. 32-36.

14. Oregon Hospice Association. OHA Supports Ballot Measure 51. 1997.

Chapter 7

Massage as Respite:

Caring for the Caregivers

Robert was my first massage patient at OHSU. He had been in the hospital for weeks and more than anything was bored. For him the massage was a pleasant distraction and something new in an otherwise dull day. He enjoyed the session well enough. His wife Sharon was my second patient. Even though she was not the "designated" patient, Sharon needed care as much, if not more, than Robert. The couple lived on a small farm near the Oregon coast. When Robert became ill with leukemia, Sharon had to do the bulk of the farm and house chores as well as maintain a part-time job. The physical and emotional burden was staggering. Driving 180 miles round trip to the hospital, feeding livestock, and parenting two sons on top of her regular responsibilities had taken a toll on her body, especially the back and shoulders. For Sharon, the neck and shoulder massage was more than a diversion, it gave her time to rest for a moment, to stop and take a few breaths.

Caring for a seriously ill family member is emotionally and physically exhausting. Caregivers are required to perform tasks for patients that are physically demanding, such as bathing, assisting

"My whole outlook changed."
— FAMILY MEMBER
OF HOSPITAL PATIENT AFTER A
15 MINUTE SEATED MASSAGE

them to the bathroom, or making transfers from the bed to a wheelchair or commode. On top of providing this extra day-to-day care, caregivers are left to manage the household chores on their own. As if all of this is not enough, they often have to rise many times during the night to attend to the patient, thereby diminishing their sleep.

Not only does the body become over-extended from the increase in duties and lack of sleep, but it becomes tense and armored due to fear, grief, and even anger. Evidence proves that this stress can suppress components of the immune system. Researchers studying wound healing in a group of female caregivers who scored high in psychological stress found that they took 24 percent longer to heal than non-caregivers who scored low on the stress test.[1] If stress decreases immune response, it could be hypothesized that interventions that decrease stress would increase the immune system. Dr. Tiffany Fields and her associates at the Touch Research Institute are finding this to be true. In studies with other stressed groups such as AIDS patients, depressed teens, and premature infants, Fields has found massage to have a positive effect on components of the immune system, such as natural killer cells, or to lower levels of the stress hormones cortisol and norepinephrine.[2,3]

Massage not only improves immune function, but it can address directly many of the stresses of caregiving: fatigue, isolation, a decreased sense of well-being, an increase in physical symptoms, insufficient personal time, and perhaps a loss of physical affection. However, many, including some health care workers, see massage as an unaffordable luxury. But, by offering services that support family caregivers directly, health care agencies and the families themselves may save money in the long run as caregiver demands on agency resources are reduced. A rested caregiver who is attending to some of her own needs will be able to provide more and better care for the patient.

THE HOSPITAL WAIT

reading all the signs
for the umpteenth time
-O.R. waiting room
— HANK DUNLAP

hospital vigil
the imperceptible shift
of clouds
— FRANCINE PORAD

After receiving the diagnosis, the first taste caregivers have of the cancer experience is often in the hospital when the patient begins treatment. Time in hospitals is characterized by endless amounts of waiting, waiting for loved ones to come out of surgery, "standing watch" for days, or even weeks, at the bedside, and enduring nights "sleeping" in a reclining chair. At the very least there are frequent day-long waits in the outpatient clinic while the patient receives chemotherapy or radiation. A short seated massage can give release to pent-up bodies and minds, provide a pleasant distraction, and allow those in the role of givers to receive, just for a moment.

When Giving Seated Massage in the Hospital to Family Caregivers:

- Observe intake protocols for giving seated massage, even if the session will only be 5 minutes. Quickly inquire about the recipient's general health, anything that might contribute to easy bruising, the condition of the skin in the areas to be worked (because the massage is through clothing the practitioner cannot assess the skin visually), and the health of the neck, shoulders, back, and arms.

- Handwash before and after each session.

- Be adaptable and flexible with regard to time, location, and necessary props. Sometimes waiting family members only have five minutes to receive massage, or must leave suddenly part way through. Be willing to conduct the session wherever the caregiver is most comfortable. Sometimes people want to leave the room for a few minutes of rest and relaxation. At other times they want to remain in the patient's room. Learn to give a massage using only a regular chair. (Figure 7-1.) Often there is only a brief window of opportunity to give a session, and the moment can instantly evaporate if the therapist needs to leave to set up a seated massage chair or to get other props. If caregivers perceive that the bodyworker is going to a lot of trouble on their account, they will sometimes suddenly decline the opportunity.

- Suggest a neck and shoulder massage to caregivers when the practitioner and family member are both waiting for the patient to return from the lab, or to finish a session with the physical therapist, or to consult with physicians. In this situation, the caregivers feel as if they are not a bother, since the massage therapist is also waiting around. Even if the wait is only going to be four minutes long, offer to massage just the neck or just the shoulders. Any contact helps to develop rapport for the future. Many cancer patients are in and out of the hospital on a regular basis, so practitioners become familiar with them, their families, and friends. On-going relationships develop over time.

- Never pressure people to accept a massage. If the offer of bodywork is firmly turned down from the start, move on to the next potential recipient. Only offer again if caregivers are showing some ambivalence. Perhaps they need a little encouragement to do something for themselves or need to get further information about the process of seated massage. Oftentimes caregivers may initially act excited at the prospect of receiving some T.L.C. and then just as suddenly will back away with a comment such as, "I was just kidding" or, "Save your energy for the patients".

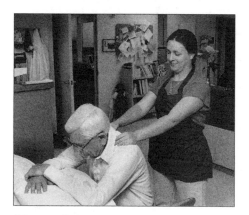

Figure 7-1.

- An unused overbed table positioned against the wall makes a good station from which to give a seated massage, especially if the caregiver wishes to remain in the loved one's room. Raise the table up to the most advantageous height and place several pillows on the top.

PROVIDING CARE AT HOME

While the hospital experience is distinguished by long periods of inactivity for care partners, caring for someone at home, whether recovering from chemotherapy or surgery, or in the last stage of life, is characterized by running from morning until night. Accepting support for themselves can be difficult for family care providers. They feel there isn't enough time, or if they relax they may never get back up. Some feel guilty receiving TLC for themselves when their loved one is sick or dying.

Marti, a friend of mine who is a massage therapist, was the primary caregiver for her dying grandmother. She related that during the time she cared for her grandmother, she never had a massage for fear of falling apart. Marti was certain if she received a massage she would not be able to "hold it together" and would be unable to fulfill her responsibilities to her grandmother and her sons.

Caregivers may need to be encouraged and helped in learning to take time for themselves. They often don't understand that by taking care of themselves they can better take care of the patient. Bodyworkers, however, can only offer their skills as a way of helping family caregivers. If the caregiver's decision is "No," practitioners must accept it without exerting pressure. Other ways can be found to give support, such as staying with the patient while the primary caregiver (PCG) goes out or by doing the grocery shopping. The massage therapist can let her know the offer is always there if she changes her mind. Very few families can afford to pay for extras such as massage during a serious illness. Even with good insurance coverage, the out-of-pocket expenses are financially depleting. Professional practitioners must bear this in mind when offering massage.

HOSPICE CAREGIVERS

Caring for a family member at home who is at the end stage of life is particularly demanding for primary caregivers. Some families provide all of the care themselves without the help of a hospice agency. But even with the assistance of a hospice program, the task for caregivers is overwhelming. Those unfamiliar with hospice care may erroneously think that the hospice agency provides the day-to-day nursing care, but it is usually a member of the patient's family who does this. The hospice team is there to make home visits, monitor medications, coordinate professional and volunteer caregivers, instruct family members in patient care, plus many other services. It

Caregivers... may sense that letting themselves be nurtured and cared for will make them feel vulnerable or bring up feelings that they are reluctant to face or accept. It is important to acknowledge and accept such fears or reluctance and not to challenge someone to move beyond what they feel they are capable of.

— DAWN NELSON,
Compassionate Touch

is the PCG who performs the tasks of daily living, such as bathing, oral hygiene, special skin care, preparation of special meals, bowel care, assisting to the bathroom, or helping with exercise regimens. Caregivers often must learn special procedures to care for catheters or colostomies, to monitor IVs, or to keep track of the patient's fluid intake and output.

Successful hospice care is dependent on a caregiver who is willing and able to attend to the needs of the dying loved one 24 hours a day, with infrequent help from the hospice agency. Generally, hospice care is begun when the physician feels that the patient has six months or less to live. However, it is likely that the PCG has been attending to her loved one throughout the illness, so that by the time hospice care is begun, she will already be mentally, emotionally, and physically exhausted. Caregiver fatigue is one of the main deterrents to successful hospice intervention and is a fundamental reason why patients must be institutionalized in the final phases of their illness.

The majority of hospice patients are over 65, so caregivers, too, are often in advanced years, with health problems of their own. One survey of a midwest hospice organization found that "the frail elderly individual is the most common problem regarding family caregivers."[4] Spousal caregivers, who comprise the bulk of hospice care partners, have been found to experience increased symptoms, and a decreased sense of well-being before and after the death of the ill spouse.[5] Other stresses are isolation, lack of time for themselves,[6] the loss of physical affection from the dying loved one,[5] and the need to be more socially active.[7]

Supporting caregivers is highly beneficial during this arduous time. The average hospice patient spends eight of his last 50 days in the hospital.[8] A patient with an exhausted caregiver is likely to spend more than the eight days or is more likely to be permanently transferred to a care facility, and is less likely to die at home. Therefore, directly caring for the PCG is beneficial not only to the patient, but to the providing agency, and in the long run to society through reduced health care costs.

Massage as Respite

Cancer doesn't just happen to one person, but to the entire family. The hospice philosophy recognizes this, and sees the "unit of care" as not just the person with the symptoms, but the family too. However, despite including the family in the unit of care, most of the direct care is still focused on patients. PCGs often express a desire for direct support "rather than being instructed about how to attain it through self-reliant means."[5]

Respite care is one way hospice programs provide for the needs of caregivers. Typically when a respite volunteer comes in for a few hours, it allows the PCG a chance to get out on errands, shop, or to

Caregivers commonly take on more than they need to – and often more than the person receiving care wants them to.

— JEAN DUNN,
LONG TERM CARE
RESOURCE MANAGER

[One of] the... most important things caregivers should do is pay attention to their own health. There is such a clear association between the stress a caregiver feels and the quality of care the patient receives, that stress management is vital.

— KEN BRUMMEL-SMITH, M.D.

keep an appointment. However, a pilot outreach program through the Oregon Hospice Association successfully used massage as a respite intervention. Massage therapists traveled with their tables to the recipients's home, which made it easier for the PCGs to participate in the program. Participants received a series of full-body massages, usually weekly or bi-weekly. On average, six massages were given in the series, although some received only three sessions, while a few received up to eight. The majority of recipients were women who were caring for male loved ones. Their ages ranged from 35 – 82, with nearly half being over 70. About half had never had a massage.

EDGAR

Edgar, 82 years old, is a sweet, soft, gentle man who is just about spent emotionally and physically. He has been caring for his wife Maureen, who is in the end stage of metastatic breast cancer to the lung, for several months. Taking care of her as well as maintaining the house and yard are overwhelming. He rated his emotional and physical stress at 4 and 4.5 respectively on a 1-5 scale, with 1 being low and 5 being high.

After the last time Maureen returned home from the hospital, stress fractures occurred at T10 – L4. Edgar feels they are a result of his emotional distress. The fractures cause him a lot of pain and make it difficult to lift and position Maureen, even though she only weighs 58 pounds. He rated his physical pain at a 5. Sleep too is difficult, which he rated at a 4. Every two to three hours he must rise to help Maureen. Usually Edgar sleeps until three A.M. and lays awake until it's time to get up. He just hired a caregiver because he is only able manage now until two P.M.

WEEK 1. Because of the back pain, Edgar asked me to focus on that area as well as general relaxation. I used Swedish and Russian effleurage, petrissage, and friction, as well as gentle vibration and shaking to the shoulders, back, and gluteals. His pain didn't seen to be in the spine but in the left quadratus lumborum (QL). The new caregiver also had massaged the area, leaving it bruised and sore. Edgar reported that, "She really went after that spot!" I will show her how to work the area next week when I come.

WEEK 2. Edgar seems less stressed and his back is better. The hired caregiver and massage are helping a lot. I used Muscle Energy Technique to stretch and release the QL, as well as applying relaxation strokes.

WEEK 3. Maureen's son is visiting. He is here to make the final arrangements and yet talks as if his mother will recover. Edgar is sleeping better and his sense of humor is surfacing. Unless he lifts something, his back is all right. As I left, Maureen's parting comment was that she probably wouldn't be here next week.

WEEK 4. Maureen was asleep when I arrived. Edgar's daughter is visiting, which noticeably raised his spirits. She is a massage therapist in California, so I showed her what I've been doing with her father's back. Edgar's back continues to improve, but he forgets to put on the back support when helping Marie into and out of bed, which makes his back hurt.

The project's primary objective was to reduce the fatigue and stress that compromise the PCG's ability to effectively care for the dying loved one at home. Feedback given at the end of the series of massages indicated that this objective was met for every caregiver but one. Data was collected prior to starting the series of massages and following the final session on four items: emotional stress, physical stress, physical pain, and sleep difficulties. A decrease in emotional and physical stress was reported by 85 percent of the participants (n=13). Physical pain, which was defined as specific symptoms such as headaches, back pain, or pain from knotted or strained muscles, decreased in 77 percent of the group. Sleep difficulties were reduced for 54 percent.

WEEK 5. A couple of days ago Maureen fell during the night. Her cries for help eventually woke Edgar. He tried to help her up but couldn't, and hurt his back again. Together they crawled to the bed so Maureen could help pull herself up. He was especially glad to see me today, the back problem is really getting him down. I focused on the lower back from T10-L4. He soaked up the massage. Tomorrow Edgar leaves for a week to see his brother and is expecting flak from the family. He needs to get away from Maureen. Her anger and attitude is getting to him.

WEEK 6. Maureen is in great pain owing to muscle spasms from coughing. Edgar looks refreshed from his week away. The focus was on full-body relaxation.

WEEK 7. The house was quiet today. Maureen continues to be in pain from muscles spasms, but was asleep at the time. Edgar seemed in a good space today. I thing he looks forward to the massage so much he automatically feels better on these days. His back is good. There were no situations this past week to stress or reinjure it. The massage session focused on the low back and shoulders. He always tells me, "I'll give you 24 hours to stop". We talked about how much better his back feels now and how grateful he is.

WEEK 8. Maureen is still having a lot of pain. She hurts too much to be touched and is on morphine now. Edgar is stressed again this week. The hospice nurse had been there just before my visit to teach him how to administer morphine injections. Since this was his last massage as part of the Massage Respite Project, he asked for "one more good back massage". Since starting, his back is much better overall. Unless he does something to stress it, he is pain free. Before starting the series of eight massages, his physical pain was a 5. By the end of the series it had dropped to a 2. Edgar's emotional stress also dropped from a 4 to a 2, physical stress from 4.5 to a 2, and sleep difficulties went from a 4 to a 2. Thanks to the massages he was better able to care for his wife.

— *Courtesy of the Massage Respite Project*

Typical responses were, "The massages have been extraordinarily helpful. They were very successful in relieving built-up stress." A.M., a 71 year old woman wrote, "I am sad the massages are almost over. I really looked forward to them each week and it's a good way to relieve physical and emotional stress. It is also very good therapy for the spirit." Before receiving any massages, R.B., a 74 year old caring for her husband reported "having some really bad days lately – no one left to share the burden." Following a series of eight massages, R.B. wrote, "I am more relaxed. I still have much tension, but it seems easier to handle at times. I find I don't have to do everything right now, it'll still be there." S.K., a 35 year old woman who cared for her mother in addition to her own family, reported "I am surprised at how much the massages helped. I didn't think they would. They helped me realize where I carry my stress – the headaches are gone, and muscles are not tight."

Only one caregiver did not notice any long term benefits from the three massages he received. Each massage felt great to him while it was happening and immediately following, but it was very difficult to return to the same stressful situation afterwards. Most of the relaxation was gone as soon as he left the room. This was one of the few PCGs to complete at least three massages who was also working full-time. The added stress of working and caring for his wife no doubt contributed to his incredibly high stress level. On the whole, a series of massages was not a successful intervention for caregivers who were also working full-time. Originally the idea sounded good to them, but their day was already so full that one more thing couldn't be squeezed in without it being an added stress. Most discontinued after one or two sessions. The greatest benefit was to those who were full-time caregivers.

SUPPORT DURING THE DYING PROCESS

As the patient enters the active stages of dying, the experience intensifies for the caregiver. During the final stages they may react with physical symptoms, such as headaches, fatigue, loss of appetite, insomnia, and muscular tension; and with such emotional symptoms as fear, guilt, anger, depression, sorrow, relief, withdrawal, or peace.[9] Care partners may need encouragement to take some time for themselves. A walk, a nap, hot bath, or seated massage can help them preserve the energy and composure needed to sustain care for the dying loved one as well as maintain a calm environment. (Figure 7-2)

Vicky, whose 82 year-old father was dying in the hospital, was very distraught by her father's struggle to breathe. As the massage students were debriefing, his nurse put her head in the conference room and asked if someone would do an "emergency massage" for this man. Pam volunteered. When she entered the room, the patient was having difficulty breathing. His daughter felt he should rest and was not in favor of her father being massaged. Pam gently asked if she could just hold the patient's feet, which Vicky consented to. At first he gave a

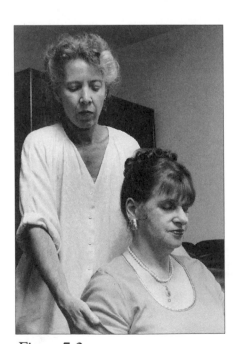

Figure 7-2.

couple of twitches and jerks. Pam thought he might die at that moment, but within five minutes, his breathing calmed, along with the atmosphere in the room. Soon after, Pam gave the distressed daughter a seated massage in another room, enabling her to relax. The patient died the following day. The charge nurse reported that everyone was calmer that final day. It will never be known to what extent Pam's ministrations were helpful, but perhaps the massage played some part in making a painful situation more bearable.

Another family was momentarily transformed by the soothing effects of massage as they struggled to endure the discomfort of the dying man who was their brother, son, and husband. As the night wore on, different family members would leave the hospital room and wander the halls, the despair evident on their faces. In some miraculous way, each of those four people independently found their way to one of the massage students who has just started their first night of work on the oncology unit. When the students' evening ended, they all passed by the patient's room on their way back to the debriefing room. The entire family, who was relaxed and smiling, came out to thank the students for their care. Allowing themselves to be massaged for just 15 minutes had palpably shifted the mood from anguish to tranquility.

I noticed my mood changed after each massage. I could face the world a little better. It was easier to go back and tackle things.

**— K.C.,
42 year-old woman
who cared for her brother**

Easing the Way During Bereavement

Often during the Massage Respite Project, the patient died before the caregiver had received all of the massages in the series. The sessions then became part of the bereavement process. One 56 year old participant, who received a series of three massage, all after her husband's death, wrote, "It gave me something to look forward to and helped relieve the stress during this hard time. It was so nice to be taken care of after so many months of taking care of others." One of the most touching stories was that of a 68 year old woman who anxiously asked the nurse, almost immediately after her husband died, if she would still be given the remainder of her massages. The caregiver was afraid that after her husband died she would no longer be eligible to participate in the Project.

Not only is caregiving deleterious to the PCG's health, but so is the grieving process. The stress of bereavement has been shown to have a negative effect on components of the immune system. Calabrese et al.[10], in their review of literature in "Alterations in Immunocompetence During Stress, Bereavement, and Depression," cited studies of spouses with seriously ill partners in which the T lymphocyte responses were adversely affected. Six weeks after the partners' deaths the lymphocyte responses were even lower than at the first sampling, leading researchers to suggest a "cumulative, time-dependent effect." Another study found reduced lymphocyte response in bereaved subjects who had scored high on a depression rating scale. A study of subjects that scored high on a loneliness scale exhibited decreased immunocompetence, a relevant finding related to grieving caregivers, as loneliness is one of the stresses reported by PCGs.[10] In addition, Barasch states that "Men who suffered the loss of a spouse from breast cancer were shown to display suppressed immunity for up to two years."[11]

As was reported at the beginning of the chapter, massage has been found to have a positive influence on immune function. Although no research has been done yet to assess the immunological effect of massage on those in mourning, it is reasonable to speculate that receiving nurturing touch will be beneficial to caregivers' immune systems as they grieve the death of their spouse, child, lover, parent, or friend. A pilot study that examined the effect of Therapeutic Touch on four people who recently lost a loved one found that modality provided promising results on various immunological and psychological factors. The immune functions studied presented no consistent findings with the exception of lowered suppressor T cells in all four subjects. The function of these suppressor T cells, which is a type of lymphocyte, is to turn off the immune system. By lowering the percentage of these cells, the immune system should function at a higher level.[12]

The most dramatic results of the Therapeutic Touch study were on a psychological scale measuring positive qualities such as joy, vigor, contentment, and affection, and negative elements such as anxiety, guilt, hostility, and depression. The recipients showed significant

LUCY

Lucy's husband Joe had been in the hospice program off and on since he was diagnosed with prostate cancer two years ago. A month ago he broke his hip during a three-day stay in a nursing home and is completely bedridden. Now Lucy is no longer willing to have him cared for anywhere but home, which places an immense physical stress on her. At 69 years old, she "runs up and down the stairs all day long". Not only does he have a broken hip, but recently suffered two strokes and is quite demanding. Two weeks ago she strained her back turning Joe over in bed, which, along with arthritis in the neck and shoulders, causes much physical pain. Prior to starting the series of massages Lucy rated her physical pain at the highest possible rating, 5, with 1 being the lowest rating. She also rated her emotional stress at a 5, with physical stress at a 3, and sleep difficulties at a 2.

WEEK 1. Lucy expressed a desire for a general relaxation massage with extra attention to the back, neck, and shoulders. Turning from front to back was painful. Next week I'll work with her in side-lying position. Despite the discomfort caused from turning, Lucy reported the back pain had lessened and she "felt like a new woman." An aide comes in several times a week to help with Joe's care. We arranged our session so that the aide will be here both during and after the session so Lucy can take a nap.

WEEK 2. Lucy and Joe's daughter is visiting for a week, allowing Lucy more time to rest. Her back is still a problem, but somewhat better. I concentrated on her back using effleurage, friction, compression, and jostling. The side-lying position worked better.

WEEK 3. Lucy's back is feeling better and she's been able to rest more. Today she was able to change positions without pain. I asked how she was feeling about the massage sessions. She said, "Delighted!"

increases in the positive characteristics and marked decreases in the negative ones. However, on another inventory which just surveyed anxiety, only two of the recipients had less anxiety, while the other two had more anxiety following the series of sessions. The researchers were at a loss to explain this.[12] However, a similar occurrence happened to bereaved participants in the Massage Respite Project with regard to sleep. After the death of their loved one, some, who had been sleeping fairly well, reported increased sleep difficulties even though they were still receiving bodywork. The caregivers attributed this to the stress of adjusting to their new situation.

Evidence exists that those who care for a dying loved one at home over a long period of time find it more difficult to readjust during the early months following the death.[13] One of the primary needs during this time, if not the primary need, is for emotional support. According to Stetz and Hanson's study of caregiving demands during and after the experience, ".... a primary intervention would be to assist the caregiver emotionally with his or her grieving."[5] As Lucy's story below affirms, massage is beneficial in times of grief. Bodies that have become armored over the months and years are loosened and softened, allowing grief to move through with greater ease and speed.

People derive emotional support from a variety of avenues. For some, the deepest comfort comes from the patient's nurse, for others it is provided by the clergy or a social worker, while still others depend on family, friends, or even nature. Bodywork can be an equally viable

Grief is a sacred wound.

— Charles Durning,
1997 National Memorial Day
Concert

When she feels stressed or uncomfortable, Lucy said she has been imagining our massage sessions. This image is enough to relax her and provide relief from the tension.

WEEK 4. Joe died since the last massage. The house is quiet without the housekeeper and hospice workers coming and going. Lucy is doing fairly well. She experiences ups and downs and "moments that catch her off guard." The improvement in her back has held up through the stress. We focused on relaxation today, using Swedish Massage strokes and ending with Reiki to the face and head. I think the massage is helping her to cope with the changes in her life.

WEEK 5. Lucy has been going through old pictures and souvenirs, which brought up many memories. Sleeping has been difficult and her emotions vacillate. She is worried about now being responsible for tasks that Joe formerly took charge of, such as the bills, property taxes, and decisions regarding the house. Oddly enough, she seems more tense now than when she was caring for her husband. After the Massage Respite Project ends, she is going to continue with the massages. Relaxation was the focus of the bodywork.

WEEK 6. Lucy continues to do well. She slept better for a night or two following last week's massage. This was her final session as part of the project. Afterward she wrote, "My massages have been wonderful. I was in extreme stress both physically and emotionally. I feel these massages helped me back to being a fairly normal person again. The sessions after Joe's death may have been more important than the sessions beforehand." Before starting the series of sessions, Lucy rated her emotional stress at a 5. When the series ended she perceived it to be a 3. Physical stress dropped from a 3 to a 1, physical pain from a 5 to a 2, and sleep difficulties stayed the same at a 2.

— *Courtesy of the Massage Respite Project*

source. During a massage the caregiver is not only able to rest and be physically cared for, but is simultaneously able to tell her story to a compassionate listener. Grief is never just an emotional process; a physical component is always involved. In order to truly assist the bereaved, hospice and home health care agencies should make a diverse and holistic group of support services available, including methods that integrate the body into the process.

RECOMMENDATIONS FOR GIVING BODYWORK TO CAREGIVERS AT HOME

- Being able to receive massage in the home is important. Many hospice caregivers are reluctant to leave, even for awhile, in case something should happen to the patient.

- Put aside any preconceived notions about who would be open to receiving bodywork. Sometimes it is assumed that because of age, gender, weight, or religious conviction, a PCG would be opposed to such an opportunity. Predicting who would like to receive massage is impossible.

- Because many caregivers are in advanced years, with health problems of their own, it may be helpful to have them fill out a health history prior to the first session in case the person's physician needs to be contacted for approval or information.

- A seated massage can be an effective first session for some care partners. This allows those who have never received bodywork to ease into both the process and the relationship with the practitioner. Others are immediately ready for a full-body session. Sound out the caregiver on which would be more comfortable for her.

- Ascertain whether the patient can be left unattended for the hour it will take for the session. If constant care is required, encourage the PCG to arrange for another family member, friend, or neighbor to come to the house. This will make it possible for the caregiver to relax, knowing he will not have to get off of the table midway to help the patient.

- Call to confirm 24 hours before the session is scheduled and then call again the morning of the appointment to reconfirm. The situation can change drastically from one hour to the next when someone is seriously ill, and time can cease to exist.

FINAL THOUGHTS

The hospice model should be the universal standard of care in all situations of serious illness, not just for those families affected by a terminal disease. But even the hospice model needs expanding where caregivers are concerned. Hopefully the hospice and home health care team of the future will include a massage therapist. Bodywork practitioners bring unique skills and qualities to a health care staff. Not only do they have the training to work with sore muscles or stiff necks, touch professionals bring with them qualities such as restfulness, tranquility, deep compassion, and the ability to listen with their entire being. Through their hands these attributes are transmitted, momentarily easing the burden, nourishing the caregiver's body, mind, and heart.

Providing nurturing bodywork for care partners not only supports them, but can have an indirect benefit for patients. Caregivers, family members, or friends who have been massaged are often then able to give compassionate, loving touch to the patient. Once they have personally experienced the sensations of increased physical and emotional well-being, and become familiar with the types of strokes, the depth of pressure, and pacing, some feel confident to carry this experience over to the patient.

ACKNOWLEDGMENT

Parts of this chapter originally appeared in *Alternative Therapies in Clinical Practice*, May/June1997 and were reprinted in *The American Journal of Hospice and Palliative Care*, January/February 1998.

REFERENCES

1. Kiecolt-Glaser, J.K.; P.T. Marucha; W.B. Malarkey; A.M. Mercado; and R. Glaser. Slowing of Wound Healing by Psychological Stress. *Lancet.* 1995; 346(8984): 1194-1196.

2. Knaster, M. Premature Infants Grow with Massage. Dr. Tiffany Field's Research. *Massage Therapy Journal.* 1991; 30(3): 50-60.

3. Touch Research Institute Studies. *Hospital-Based Massage Newsletter.* 1997; 3(1): 15-19.

4. Smith, M.A. Primary Caregiver Options in Hospice Care. *American Journal of Hospice and Palliative Care.* 1994; 11(3): 15-17.

5. Stetz, K. and W. Hanson. Alterations in Perceptions of Caregiving Demands in Advanced Cancer During and After the Experience. *The Hospice Journal.* 1992; 8(3): 2-34.

6. Hull, M. Sources of Stress for Hospice Caregiving Families. *The Hospice Journal.* 1990; 6 (2): 29-54.

7. Martens, N. and B. Davis. The Work of Patients and Spouses in Managing Advanced Cancer at Home. *The Hospice Journal.* 1990; 6(2): 55-73.

8. Schapira, D.V.; J. Studnicki; and D. Bradham. Intensive Care, Survival, and Expense of Treating Critically Ill Cancer Patients. *Journal of the American Medical Association.* 1993; 269(6): 783-786.

9. Bernard, J. S. and M. Schneider. *The True Work of Dying.* New York: Avon Books, 1996.

10. Calabrese, J.R.; M.A. Kling; and P.W. Gold. Alterations in Immunocompetence During Stress, Bereavement, and Depression: Focus on Neuroendocrine Regulation. *The American Journal of Psychiatry.* 1987; 144(9): 1123-1134.

11. Barasch, M. *The Healing Path.* New York: Arkana, 1993.

12. Quinn, J.F. and A.J. Strelkaukas. Psychoimmunologic Effects of Therapeutic Touch on Practitioners and Recently Bereaved Recipients: A Pilot Study. *Advances in Nursing Science.* 1993; 15(4): 13-26.

13. Kirschling, J.M.; V.P. Tilden; and P.G. Butterfield. Social Support: The Experience of Hospice Family Caregivers. *The Hospice Journal.* 1990; 6(2): 75-93.

Chapter 8

Companions on the Journey:

Who Gives? Who Receives?

The knowledge practitioners bring to their work is, without a doubt, a vital ingredient. Understanding how cancer arises and spreads, cognizance of the research, and familiarity with indications and contraindications is important. But, the single most important resource practitioners bring to the experience is themselves. More significant than which massage techniques are in their repertoire, or their knowledge of the disease process, is therapists' way of being, who they are in relationship to themselves and those who are ill. To be sure, it is necessary to hone hands-on skill, to attend to safety precautions, and to increase understanding of medical procedures, but even more important is that touch therapists explore their motivations, attend to their heart and soul, and clarify their approach and purpose. After all, massage is not only performed with the hands, but with the entire being.

One of the criticisms of allopathic health care is that it operates from a dualistic perspective that splits body from mind, heart, and soul. This model not only separates the patient's psyche and soma, but creates divisions between staff and patients, and between staff members. In this paradigm the ill are in need, broken, and unproductive. As givers, producers, and healers, caretakers are in a

You reach someone by being within yourself.
— ROBERTA DELONG MILLER,
PSYCHIC MASSAGE

dominant position rather than being equal partners. This dualism is also evident among health care workers. On the surface, a medical staff can appear to be caring for patients as a team, but underneath, a clear pecking order is at work, and wide schisms exist.

Although bodywork is potentially one of the ultimate holistic modalities, without a conscious effort its training and method of practice can be as dualistic as the medical model. The bodyworker can just as easily take on the attitude of fixer-upper, of delineating between giver and taker, sick and well. In a holistic relationship, therapist and patient are equal partners, their journeys inextricably woven together. Each participant is allowed to assume a variety roles, therapist, patient, giver, receiver, healed, or ailing.

Not only does wholeness need to be created between the therapist and patient, but it must happen within the therapist as well. If bodyworkers are to provide a holistic experience, they must be a microcosm of it. All of the self must be brought to the encounter, not just the parts that are energetic, cheerful, serene, or healthy, but also those that are tired, depressed, confused, or wounded.

YEARNINGS OF THE SOUL

A life-threatening illness that happens to someone close to us, takes us into the underworld as a companion on the journey, and inasmuch as it will take us into our own depths of feeling and meaning, there are consequences for us as well.

— JEAN SHINODA BOLEN,
CLOSE TO THE BONE

Bodyworkers are drawn to work with different groups. Some have an affinity for athletes, others for the elderly, and those reading this book possibly feel an inclination toward cancer patients or the seriously ill. The journey each therapist embarks on becomes intertwined with that of the ill person. Together the two are initiated into the inexplicable mysteries of life and death.

Practitioners are attracted to certain groups by a complex set of motivations, many which they are conscious of, while others lie well below the surface. Some people are drawn to be with the seriously ill as a means of healing their own grief about the death of a loved one. For others it is part of a spiritual passage or the quest for a deeper and more meaningful life. It is essential that therapists reflect on the conscious and unconscious reasons for the work they do. Through this exploration fuller access to deeper capacities and special innate gifts is gained, which benefits patients in the end.

The most conscious motivation is the desire to help. Each time a new hospital massage class starts I ask the students why they want to work with cancer patients. The most common answers are — to ease the physical pain, to transform hospitals into caring places, or to be a soothing, nurturing presence. The students' focus is on what they have to give. But as soon as the work with patients begins, they realize how much there is to receive. It is they who are transformed and healed. One nurse colleague is fond of telling first-day students that after being on a cancer unit their lives will never be the same. Although the initial focus is on what we want to give, I suspect we long to receive just as much. It is important to acknowledge that we do this work for ourselves as much as for the patients. Although our work with people who are seriously ill starts out of a desire to help others, we keep coming back for us.

My dreams seem to be coming into play with whatever it is that is trying to break through in my life right now. I dreamed about being in a hospital, walking through long halls, seeing patients, while feeling and being told that there was no way I could help them. I felt the frustration for days after the dream. My whole life I've wanted to serve, to help, and in the past I haven't always felt that I could make any difference. It's all connected, my feelings about myself, helping myself, and being able to help others. I've been questioning everything in my life – my beliefs, who I am, what my life is all about. The night before going to the hospital, I felt anxious. Would I be able to make a difference? Is this my path? My head was spinning with questions. I went to sleep and the sweetest, simplest dream. I was a child on a big swing, going back and forth, free, my legs kicking, hair flying. Over and over I heard the same words – ONLY LOVE, ONLY LOVE, ONLY LOVE. Sounds kind of corny, but it make me feel wonderful! It reminded me that it is that simple. My intent now is to give love and to serve, helping myself as well as others. I feel like this whole experience is some kind of resolution to a learning that has been on-going for years. It's not done, but something major has happened. My perspective has changed. I have changed. This life is as much about my healing as it is about others. Finally I feel the importance of my own healing being the key to helping others.

— DIANE HUTSON, L.M.T.

The novelist Isabelle Allende commented that she uses writing to explore her soul. Are we exploring something in our souls by working with cancer patients? Why would it be healing or soulful to give bodywork to cancer patients? Are there qualities within their experience that we yearn for in our own lives? When we are with the ill, are we able to let certain qualities surface that aren't normally experienced?

Serious illness brings with it a new way of being in the world, a new identity, qualities often not cultivated during times of health, such as quietude, stillness, dependency, or "being" rather than "doing". The focus turns inward, masks are stripped away, we need tenderness from ourselves and others, self-worth can no longer be measured by what we produce in the world. We are forced to find new answers to the question – "Who am I?" Perhaps it is this way of being that some bodyworkers yearn for and are exploring through their work with cancer patients.

During a lecture, Thomas Moore, author of *Care of the Soul*, was asked what ideas he had to make our culture more soulful. His answer was that we need to integrate two groups more fully into our culture — children and the ill. In order to integrate illness into the culture we must first bring it into ourselves.

CHAPTER 8
COMPANIONS ON THE JOURNEY: WHO GIVES? WHO RECEIVES?

139

People who have been through illness's dark passage can occasionally give us a glimpse not only of what it is like to become whole, but of what it is to be more fully human.

— MARC IAN BARASCH,
THE HEALING PATH

After many months of massaging hospitalized cancer patients I was partially able to put my finger on why I yearn to work in this arena. Through my eyes, the experience of cancer put these people closer to God. Being in their presence brought my own longing for the divine closer to the surface. The question then was, "How can I integrate this energy into my day-to-day life?"

— G.M.

EXERCISE 1: EXPLORING THE QUALITIES OF ILLNESS

Take a moment to explore the experience of illness. Put down the book. Close your eyes. Imagine you are deeply ill. Sink into the physical sensations of being sick. Notice your energy, strength or weakness, whether you are heavy or light, still or agitated. Which feelings surface in this state of being? Are there moments of fear? Of joy? Frustration? Satisfaction? How do you view the world from this position? Let these sensations unfold for several moments, allowing in everything, pushing away nothing.

Return now to your immediate health status. Were there any of these qualities that you would like to integrate into your present life? Perhaps you would bring back the quality of softness, increased vulnerability, slowness, or less ambition? When we open to the experience of illness we see the opportunities within it, and no longer see the ill as victims to be pitied.

EXERCISE 2: WHO ARE YOU IN THE PRESENCE OF THE ILL?

Imagine a setting where you are with someone who is sick. Notice how you greet them. As you are with them, what is your demeanor? Happy? Fearful? Calm? Grateful? Pitying? Now move your attention to your body. What sensations are discernible? Are you relaxed? Tense? Open? Closed? Does your physical energy concentrate in any certain place?

Does this setting bring out parts of your being not normally in evidence? Does it allow you to experience yourself in a different way? Are there any of these qualities that you would like to take with you from this world and integrate into other worlds, such as work, family, or friends?

When Valeri imagined being in the presence of someone who is ill she no longer felt a need to have all of the answers, her stomach was calm, and she could just "be." Cliff felt less judged. Michelle was calmer and moved more slowly, and Carol was more gracious and full of humor. Being with someone who is ill moved me to greater tenderness; my heart radiated a golden light that enveloped my chest, shoulders, and head. What would it be like to bring that tenderness and radiant light into the relationships with my family, friends, and students? I shall start by trying to "teach with a radiant heart."

— G.M.

EQUAL PARTNERS

CHAPTER 8
COMPANIONS ON THE JOURNEY:
WHO GIVES? WHO RECEIVES?

141

Why take the time and effort to dive below the surface and examine the less conscious needs that motivate us to work with cancer patients? Isn't it enough to just want to help others, to ease their discomfort? This is a noble stance from which to work, but it is a one-way dynamic; the relationship between practitioner and patient is linear, with the practitioner on top and the patient on the bottom. The person who is sick is in the position of receiver, taker, needy, or broken, qualities that have less value in our culture than those of being useful, giving, strong, healthy, and energetic. Wanting to help or comfort is a good starting point, but bodyworkers must go deeper into their motivations. This is the only way to have a complete, whole relationship.

Maureen Redl writes in the *Noetic Sciences Review* (Fall 1995):

> *Many of us, especially those in health related work, think of ourselves as helpers. We call ourselves caregivers, or caretakers. The very words suggest a hierarchy of need, variation in the degrees of wellness, as well as differing abilities to fix what isn't working. To be in a position of being able to "give" care, to be a health "provider," clearly is a one-up position. Few of us call ourselves servants. Indeed, that would not be a one-up position.*

Seriously ill people often need constant care or assistance, but feel guilty to ask for what they want or need because there is no way for them to reciprocate. What a relief it would be to feel that they and their situation had something to offer the able-bodied or healthy. One day at the hospital I spotted Cheryl, an old college acquaintance, visiting a sick friend, Nancy. We stood at the foot of her bed and caught up on the last 20 years. When she discovered that I was a massage therapist, Nancy piped up and said," Oh, you can practice on me". I told her that I didn't need to practice any more, that giving massage was my purpose for being at the hospital, and I would be glad to give her one. "That's OK," she said, "I was just kidding, I'm fine." My acquaintance tried to convince her to accept the offer, "She really wants one, but is afraid to admit it," Cheryl said with a wink. We got into a three-way discussion about imposing on people. During all this, Nancy was having the hiccups, which is painful with a fresh surgical incision in the chest. Her usual ritual for getting rid of them was to stretch her arms high above her head, which she was not able to do. Every hiccup was a jolt of pain. Naturally I was curious if massage would help and Nancy seemed interested to try. We all continued chatting, including her nurse, while I gently worked her feet. Within 5–10 minutes we realized the hiccups were gone, and joked about writing a paper and applying for grant monies to study the effects of massage on hiccups.

Our service serves us as well as others. That which uses us strengthens us. Over time, fixing and helping are draining, depleting. Over time we burn out. Service is renewing. When we serve, our work itself will sustain us.

— RACHEL NAOMI REMEN, M.D.

Acting and giving are not necessarily more useful than resting and receiving.

— WAYNE MULLER

Figure 8-1. Yin/Yang Symbol

When I looked back on this encounter, I saw how my own sense of self-importance wouldn't allow me to be the student, the one who was still practicing. If in the initial stage of meeting Nancy I had said, "Thank you, I would appreciate being able to practice my massage on you," she would most likely have accepted immediately. In that way Nancy could have felt that she too was helping me. I am guessing she let me massage her feet because she sensed that I wanted to know whether massage would relax her enough to dispel the hiccups. She felt that in some way she was serving me. Now, whenever anyone says, "You're a massage therapist? Do you want someone to practice on?" I say "Yes, I'd love to."

Our culture has been programmed to believe that it is better to give than receive. But there is no distinction between giver and receiver, helper and helped. When someone won't receive, there can be no giving, they are interdependent. Just as in oriental medicine where the yin sign, which represents the qualities of dark, cold, and inwardness, contains the seed of yang, the qualities of warmth, light, and outgoingness, and vice versa, giving and receiving are inherent in one another. (Figure 8-1.) By approaching patients as equal partners we see the medicine they have to offer us, we allow them to be the teacher, the caregiver, to feel useful, giving and needed. Symptoms often magically disappear, diminish, or become more tolerable when patients feel that they belong to the process. As for us, we are more whole when we can be both student and teacher, giver and taker, expert and novice. After all, healing literally means wholeness.

TELLING OUR STORIES

During a lecture, Thomas Moore said, "We can't heal anybody, we're just here to share our stories with each other, to have a conversation." Just as patients need to tell their stories, so too do those who work with them. Through the telling the experience becomes complete and whole, and we come to better understand the events of our life. Without someone to hear and understand, we feel isolated in the experience.

For a number of years I lived with just my dog. In that time I did not suffer greatly from a lack of affection, loneliness, or boredom. What I did yearn for, though, was someone to tell my stories to at the end of the day. Without someone to relate my day to, there was a void that had nothing to do with an empty house. I felt incomplete. Touch practitioners often live a solitary professional life and can suffer from the absence of colleagues with whom to interact on a regular basis. Forming alliances or mentoring relationships is important, just to have people to whom we can tell our stories.

In his book, *Care of the Soul*, Thomas Moore writes that "Storytelling is an excellent way of caring for the soul. It helps us see the themes that circle in our lives, the deep themes that tell the myths we live." He writes about an uncle who told endless stories.

CHAPTER 8
COMPANIONS ON THE JOURNEY:
WHO GIVES? WHO RECEIVES?

143

"This I now see, was his method of working the raw material of his life, his way of turning his experience round and round...Out of that incessant storytelling I know he found added depths of meaning."

The power of having someone to share with is evident in the unexpected results of Dr. David Spiegel's study of women with metastatic breast cancer. The group who attended a weekly support group, in addition to receiving their medical regimen, survived twice as long as the group who did not attend a support group. We too need a place to share our experiences, or we shall not survive.

I write a form of Japanese poetry called haiku, but had shared it infrequently. What a joy it was when someone came into my life who also enjoyed poetry. Finally there was someone to share a part of myself that had been hidden. The circuit was completed. There was someone to bear witness to who I am. As I write this I am reminded of children who beg their parent, teacher, or friend to "Watch me, watch me." Inherent in all of us is a primal need to be watched, listened to, and acknowledged.

Whether we tell our story through poetry, journaling, drawing, sculpting, or dance, the attempt takes us inside, to the deeper layers of the event. In trying to write it, draw it, or dance it, we must look closer and more keenly. The senses become more alert to our own experience and to that of our patient.

Not only do we need a chance to tell our stories, but we need the opportunity to hear the experiences of others. Through them we are taught, inspired, guided, and affirmed. Personal stories, like myths, provide guideposts for the journey that lays ahead. Our own process is quickened by listening to the experiences of others. Through them we learn what works and what to avoid. New possibilities are opened to us, as well as giving us affirmation that we are on the right track.

IDEAS FOR CREATING HOLISM

Carl Jung believed that the unconscious pulls us toward that which will be healing. It is only by delving into this area that we become whole. In order to access the deeper, unconscious parts of the self, its language must be deciphered. The unconscious can speak through dreams, yearnings, movement, stories, symbols, places, colors, or poems. The following 10 exercises will help reveal parts of the self that unknowingly reside in uncharted waters.

Healing is the integration of psyche, soma, and spirit.

— BERNIE SIEGEL, M.D.

- Keep a bodywork story journal.

- Cultivate a relationship with a bodyworker who is doing similar work. Have a regular meeting time over tea or a meal to swap stories.

- Start a monthly support group for bodyworkers with the focus on telling the stories from your work, sharing poems, or deepening awareness of the yearnings of your soul.

If you want to know yourself, be God's hands.

— DEBORAH TAYLOR

- Write a short story or case history about a patient for submission to a professional periodical or hospital newsletter.

- Set aside one day or one bodywork session where you let go of your identity as a healer or therapist. Instead, give massage as if you were the receiver, or the student, or the one in need of healing.

- Pretend you are a poet. Give touch from this poet-self.

- Assume an outlook of gratitude. Massage a patient from this place.

- Meditate on cancer. Notice the physical sensations the word evokes. Say the word "cancer" several times inside your head. Notice the tone and feelings with which you say it. If cancer were a symbol, what would it look like? Feel the energy of it in your body. Draw the symbol. Is this symbol relevant in your own life?

- Write or imagine a fairy tale about someone who has a gift for using touch to comfort the ill. What is the setting of the story? When does it take place? What does the central figure look like? What qualities does he possess? Imagine in detail this character giving healing touch to someone who is ill. Are there parts of this fairy tale that you wish were true for you?

- Pretend a friend or loved one has cancer. Imagine spending a few hours, or even the day, together. Hear the conversations you might have. Envision your actions. Sense your feelings. Are there ways in which you are different? What parts of this scenario would you like to integrate into your real-life relationship with this person?

Afterword

This book provides detailed answers on some topics, offers a cursory look at others, but has left many issues unexplored. *Medicine Hands* is not intended to be the final authority on administering massage to people with cancer. It is meant to put forward some fundamental, basic information, to soothe the fears of practitioners in regard to comfort-oriented bodywork, and to trigger discussion within the massage community, especially the American one. As a profession, massage therapy must educate itself, consult with oncology specialists, engage in a lengthy dialogue, and then agree on a common approach to people with cancer.

The attitudes instilled in bodyworkers during their training influence their behavior throughout their careers. Because of this, massage students should be instructed from the beginning that there is always a way to touch people who have cancer. Teaching them that cancer is a contraindication for Swedish Massage often is translated in students' minds to mean people with cancer should not be touched, period. Another common interpretation is that clients with a history of cancer, irrespective of the amount of time passed, cannot be massaged; or, that all bodywork modalities, not just Swedish Massage, are contraindicated.

Seeds should be planted in beginning massage school classes that encourage students to at least massage feet, hands, and face. As they further their education, students should be taught to adapt their pressure, to avoid certain sites, and to massage patients who may have a variety of position restrictions. The power of simple, gentle touch must be emphasized. Deep, effortful bodywork is not necessary in order to create profound effects. Deep contact is made not by what we do, but by being with the person as they undergo their experience.

Massage therapists often relate stories to me about their work with clients who have cancer. Some of these reports are preceded by a request for confidentiality and are told in a voice reserved for the confessional. "If my massage board or association knew I was working with cancer patients, I would be in big trouble," is a common preamble. The telling of the story often seems like a plea for absolution. It is unfortunate they feel guilt and the need to be secretive about performing an act that is so beneficial.

I have also been told anecdotes from the other end of the spectrum by practitioners who followed their story with the postscript, "I don't know much about working with people who have cancer, but my intentions were good, so I trusted I would do no harm." Without a doubt, intention is a powerful influence. However, it should be combined with the caution of the first storytellers as well as knowledge about the disease process and the pertinent side effects of treatment. Good intentions may not always be enough.

Because of the fear of legal liability, some American bodyworkers are averse to working with cancer patients. However, liability is the reason bodyworkers must be educated. If massage therapy is going to press for inclusion into mainstreamed health care, it must take responsibility for training its members to work with everyone. Disciplines related to massage therapy, such as physical, occupational, and respiratory therapy all provide unconditional care for those with cancer. Massage therapy must do the same. "Just saying NO" is not the solution to avoiding liability.

Medicine Hands has not addressed every topic that relates to massaging those with cancer. Some readers may have wished for information on subjects such as massaging children, charting, insurance reimbursement, or positioning patients. Others may have wanted greater detail on administering bodywork to cancer patients with lymphoma or surgical incisions. Some topics, such as touch for children, were not addressed because of lack of experience on my part. Others, such as hands-on skills, were left out because they are best learned in the presence of a teacher skilled in the techniques who also understands how to apply them for people who have cancer.

My suggestion for learning hands-on skills is to seek private tutoring or formal group instruction, accompanied by supervised, clinical experience. I often turn to registered nurses for instruction in areas in which I have no training, such as positioning patients. All nurses can be helpful for such general situations as DVT or universal precautions, but if you need advice pertaining to oncology, go to specialists in that field.

While this book does not speak to every possible issue, it does present an abundance of information, which can be overwhelming at first. After reading *Medicine Hands*, working with cancer patients may appear to be a potential mine field. These people, however, are far tougher and more resilient than we know and will not break when touched. A safe and beneficial experience can be insured if a few basic guidelines are remembered:

- Be gentle. Emphasize soothing rather than stirring up. (Use pressureless techniques for DVT and thrombocytopenia.)

- Avoid sites affected by surgery, medical devices, tumors, or skin problems.

- Observe standard and protective isolation precautions.

- Wait two months following the end of treatment and a pronouncement of remission by the doctor to initiate treatment-oriented bodywork for such conditions as adhesions, scarring, and lymphedema.

The therapist will also have a positive and energizing experience if they put their attention on:

- What can be done, instead of what can't.

- Being with the person, rather than trying to fix them.

- Receiving as well as giving.

The sophistication of Western medicine is breath-taking, but it is not the total answer to complete and comprehensive health care. Neither, however, are the age-old, natural therapies. Both are good at what they do, but alone, neither is enough. Most likely, the answer lies in a marriage of the old and the new. The medicine contained in the surgeon's hands, in the energy of radiation beams, or in drug treatments can be all the more effective when combined with the simple medicine found in the hands of every family member, friend, and practitioner who cares for someone with cancer.

Appendix A
Vocabulary
and
Medical Terminology

Following is a partial list of commonly used vocabulary and medical terminology. It is helpful to have your own medical dictionary.

ADJUVANT THERAPY   The use of another form of treatment in addition to the primary one.

ALLOGENEIC TRANSPLANT   Bone marrow donated by someone other than the patient.

ANALGESIC   Pain medication.

ANAPLASTIC   Loss of cell differentiation, a characteristic of malignant cells.

ANGIOGRAM   An X-ray of blood vessels. A dye is injected that shows up in the X-ray pictures.

ANTIBODIES   Proteins made by certain white blood cells that fight infection and disease.

ANTIEMETIC   Medication to prevent or relieve nausea or vomiting.

ASPIRATION   Removal of a sample of fluids and cells through a needle.

AUTOLOGOUS TRANSPLANT   Bone marrow donated by the patient.

BONE MARROW   The soft, spongy tissue in the center of large bones that produces white blood cells, red blood cells, and platelets.

BOLUS   In this context, it most often refers to an additional amount of a drug, usually pain medication, above and beyond the prescribed amount. It can be administered by the patient or caregiver as needed.

CACHEXIA   A state of ill health, malnutrition, and wasting.

CARCINOGEN   A cancer causing agent.

CARCINOMA IN SITU   Cancer that involves only the tissue in which it began. It has not spread to other tissues.

CATHETER   A tube used for removing or injecting fluids into body cavities.

CENTRAL LINE   A semi-permanent IV in the torso, usually the chest. Once a central line has been inserted the health care staff can draw blood, administer medications, and give chemotherapy without having to put in a new IV each time.

CENTRAL LINE IV CATHETERS (types of)
        1. Groshong 2. Hickman 3. Quinton 4. port

COLOSTOMY   The opening of some part of the colon onto the abdominal surface.

CAT SCAN (CT – COMPUTERIZED TOMOGRAPHY)

An X-ray that uses a computer to produce cross-sectional pictures of the body.

CYST

A closed sac or capsule that is filled with fluid.

CYSTECTOMY

Removal of the bladder.

DOUBLE LUMEN

Two openings (i.e., type of central line catheter).

ECTOMY

Removal of any organ or gland.

EMBOLI

A detached mass in the blood stream that may consist of bits of tissue, tumor cells, fat globules, air bubbles, clumps of bacteria, and foreign bodies.

EMESIS

Vomiting.

EPIDURAL PUMP

A method of delivering analgesia into the spinal area.

FOLEY CATHETER

Urinary tract catheter.

HYSTERECTOMY

Removal of the uterus.

Total hysterectomy – Removal of the uterus and cervix.

Radical hysterectomy – Removal of the uterus, fallopian tubes, ovaries, adjacent lymph nodes and part of the vagina.

ILEOSTOMY

The opening of some part of the lower section of the small intestine, referred to as the ileum, onto the abdominal surface.

INCONTINENCE

Inability to control the flow of urine from the bladder.

JEJUNOSTOMY

Surgical opening of some part of the middle section of the small intestine, referred to as the jejunum, onto the abdominal surface.

J-POUCH

A bag attached at the site of a jejunostomy for the purpose of collecting intestinal contents.

J.P. TUBE (JACKSON-PRATT)   A type of drain.

LAPAROSCOPY

Exploration of the organs in the abdomen in which a lighted instrument (laparoscope) is inserted through a small incision.

LAPAROTOMY

An operation to open the abdomen.

LEUKOPENIA

A low white blood cell count.

LOBECTOMY

Removal of an entire lobe of the lung.

LUMPECTOMY

Surgical removal of a tumor from the breast. No other tissue or lymph nodes are removed.

MASTECTOMY

Removal of the breast

MRI (MAGNETIC RESONANCE IMAGING)

A diagnostic test that uses a magnet linked to a computer screen to create cross sectional pictures of the body.

NEO-BLADDER

A new bladder fashioned from an inverted section of the colon.

NEPHRECTOMY

Removal of the kidney.

Appendix A-2

NEUTROPENIA	Low neutrophil count. Neutrophils are the most numerous form of white blood cells.
OOPHRECTOMY	Removal of one or both ovaries.
ORCHIECTOMY	Removal of a testicle.
OSTOMY	Surgically formed artificial opening.
PALLIATIVE	To relieve or alleviate without curing.
PERIPHERAL LINE	An IV in the lower arm.
PNEUMONECTOMY	Removal of the entire lung.
RADIATION RECALL	A reaction that occurs during chemotherapy to some people who were previously treated with radiation. Certain drugs can cause the irradiated skin to turn red, to itch, and to burn.
REFLUX	When liquid backs up into the esophagus from the stomach.
RESECTION	To cut off or out a portion of a structure or organ.
SHUNT	An artificially constructed passage to divert flow from one main route to another.
STAGE	The extent of the disease.
STEM CELLS	Primitive blood cells that grow into different components of the blood, such as red blood cells, white blood cells, and platelets. Stem cells are found in the blood and bone marrow.
THORACOTOMY	An operation to open the chest.
THROMBOCYTOPENIA	Low platelets.
THROMBOPHLEBITIS	Inflammation of a vein caused by the formation of a blood clot.
TUMOR MARKER	A substance in the blood or other body fluids that may suggest that a person has cancer.
ULTRASOUND	A test that bounces sound waves off tissues and changes the echoes into pictures. Tissue with different densities reflect sound waves differently.
UROSTOMY	The redirection of urine outside of the body after the bladder has been repaired or removed.

REFERENCE

1. Thomas, C.L., ed. *Taber's Cyclopedic Medical Dictionary*. Philadelphia: F.A. Davis Co, 1993.

Appendix B
Abbreviations

Many abbreviations are universally accepted, but others are specific to certain facilities or physicians. Each organization will have a list of abbreviations they consider "official," and some of them may be different than indicated here.

$\overline{A}$	before
ALL	acute lymphoblastic (lymphocytic) leukemia
AML	acute myeloblastic (myelocytic) leukemia
APL	acute promyelocytic leukemia
BMBx	bone marrow biopsy
BMT	bone marrow transplant
Bx	biopsy
BBBD	blood brain barrier disruption
$\overline{c}$	with
CA	cancer
CBC	complete blood count
CC	chief complaint
c/o	complains of
CLL	chronic lymphocytic leukemia
DL	double lumen (i.e., type of central line catheter)
DVT	deep vein thrombosis
Dx	diagnosis
Fx	fracture
GVHD	graft versus host disease
HD	hodgkins disease

Hx	history
HOH	hard of hearing
Ⓛ	left
mets	metastases
MUD	matched unrelated donor
NG	nasogastric
NHL	non-Hodgkins lymphoma
$\overline{P}$	post
PCA	patient controlled analgesia
PICC	peripherally inserted central catheter
plts.	platelets
prn (pro re nata)	as necessary
pt.	patient
Ⓡ	right
RUQ	right upper quadrant
LUQ	left upper quadrant
RLQ	right lower quadrant
LLQ	left lower quadrant
$\overline{s}$	without
SCD	sequential compression device
Tx	treatment
WBC	white blood count

Appendix C
Types of Cancers

The following list defines some of the more commonly encountered types of cancers.

ACUTE GRANULOCYTIC LEUKEMIA (AGL). Marked by an increase in the white blood cells called granulocytes. These cells are made in the bone marrow. This type of leukemia progresses very rapidly and most often occurs in children.

ACUTE LYMPHOCYTIC LEUKEMIA (ALL). Marked by an increased number of lymphocytes. These cells are mostly made in the lymph nodes. ALL also progresses very rapidly and most often occurs in children.

ACUTE MYELOCYTIC LEUKEMIA (AML). Another name for acute granulocytic leukemia.

ADENOCARCINOMA. A malignant adenoma that arises from a glandular organ.

ADENOMA. A neoplasm of glandular epithelium.

BASAL CELL CARCINOMA. A neoplasm that occurs in the basal cells of the skin. It has a low incidence of malignancy.

BENIGN. A non-invasive tumor.

BURKITT'S LYMPHOMA. A type of non-Hodgkins lymphoma that occurs most often in people 12-30 years old. The disease usually causes a rapidly growing tumor in the abdomen.

CANCEROUS. Pertains to malignant growth.

CARCINOMA. A new growth or malignant tumor that has it's origin in epithelial tissue.

CHONDROSARCOMA. Cancer that forms in cartilage.

CHRONIC GRANULOCYTIC LEUKEMIA (CGL). A slow progressing form of leukemia in which an abnormal number of granulocytes are produced. It most often occurs in adults.

CHRONIC LYMPHOCYTIC LEUKEMIA (CLL). Also slow progressing form in which too many lymphocytes are produced. It most often occurs in adults.

CHRONIC MYELOGENOUS LEUKEMIA (CML). Another name for chronic granulocytic leukemia.

EWINGS SARCOMA. A bone cancer that forms in the shaft of large bones, most often in the hips, thighs, and upper arm bones.

FIBROID. A benign tumor of the uterus.

GLIOBLASTOMA. A type of tumor found in the brain.

HODGKINS DISEASE (HD). HD is a type of lymphoma that is characterized by the presence of one particular cell, called the Reed-Sternberg cell. The disease tends to spread in a fairly predictable manner, moving from one part of the lymphatic system to the next, and then into related organs such as the lungs and liver.

KAPOSI'S SARCOMA (KS). A malignant neoplasm of the skin associated with AIDS.

LEUKEMIA. Excessive production of abnormal white blood cells. Leukemic cells lack the ability of normal white blood cells to fight infections.

LIPOMA. A fatty tumor.

LYMPHOMA. A general term for a neoplasm of the lymphatic system.

MALIGNANT. An invasive tumor.

MELANOMA. A malignant tumor containing dark pigment, such as a mole. It is the most dangerous of all skin cancers because of its tendency to metastasize.

METASTASES. Cancer growths that started from cancer cells in another part of the body.

METASTATIC. Cancer that has spread from the original site to a distant, secondary one.

MULTIPLE MYELOMA. Cancer of the plasma cells, a type of white blood cell found in the bone marrow. Plasma cells normally produce antibodies for the body's immune system, which are used to attack viruses and bacteria.

NEOPLASM. A new and abnormal formation of tissue which can become benign or malignant.

NEUROMA. A tumor that arises in nerve cells.

NON-HODGKINS LYMPHOMA. The most common lymphoma. The progress of this form is less systematic and predictable.

OSTEOSARCOMA. A malignant sarcoma of the bone.

POLYP. A tumor with a stem. They are often found in the nose, uterus, and rectum.

SARCOMA. Cancer that arises from connective tissue, such as muscle, cartilage, or bone.

SOFT TISSUE SARCOMA. Cancer that begins in the muscle, fat, fibrous tissue, blood vessels, or other supporting tissue of the body. It is not a type of bone cancer.

SQUAMOUS CELL CARCINOMA. A tumor that develops in the squamous cells of the skin. It can metastasize, but has a high cure rate when properly treated.

TUMOR. A spontaneous new growth of tissue that forms an abnormal mass.

REFERENCES

1. Thomas, C.L., ed. *Taber's Cyclopedic Medical Dictionary*. Philadelphia: F.A. Davis Co, 1993.

2. Booklet titled *Acute Lymphocytic Leukemia*. Leukemia Society of America. 1990.

3. Booklet titled *Chronic Lymphocytic Leukemia*. Leukemia Society of America. 1988.

4. Booklet titled *Chronic Myelogenous Leukemia*. Leukemia Society of America. 1991.

5. Booklet titled *Facts on Skin Cancer*. American Cancer Society. 1992.

6. Booklet titled *Hodgkins Disease and the Non-Hodgkin's Lymphomas*. Leukemia Society of America. 1991.

7. Booklet titled *What Everyone Should Know About Leukemia*. Leukemia Society of America. 1991.

8. Booklet titled *What You Need to Know About Multiple Myeloma*. U.S. Dept. of Health and Human Services. 1988.

Appendix D
Sample Forms

PATIENT EVALUATION OF MASSAGE EXPERIENCE

The purpose of this form is to provide feedback to the massage therapists which will assist them in their learning and to provide feedback to the hospital which will help evaluate the use of massage in patient care.

Patient: _____   Time of massage: ____:____ am pm

Massage Therapist: _____   Date: _____

BEFORE THE MASSAGE

Please circle the number that indicates your level of pain, physical and emotional comfort, and fatigue.

PAIN RATING:

Extremely Comfortable												Extremely Uncomfortable
	0	1	2	3	4	5	6	7	8	9	10	

PHYSICALLY:

Extremely Comfortable						Extremely Uncomfortable
	1	2	3	4	5	

EMOTIONALLY and/or MENTALLY:

Extremely Comfortable						Extremely Uncomfortable
	1	2	3	4	5	

FATIGUE:

No Fatigue						Severe Fatigue
	1	2	3	4	5	

AFTER THE MASSAGE

List words that describe the sensations you noticed during the massage:

_____

_____

Other comments:

_____

_____

_____

Please circle the number that indicates your level of pain, physical and emotional comfort, and fatigue.

PAIN RATING:

| Extremely Comfortable | 0 | 1 | 2 | 3 | 4 | 5 | 6 | 7 | 8 | 9 | 10 | Extremely Uncomfortable |

PHYSICALLY:

| Extremely Comfortable | 1 | 2 | 3 | 4 | 5 | Extremely Uncomfortable |

EMOTIONALLY and/or MENTALLY:

| Extremely Comfortable | 1 | 2 | 3 | 4 | 5 | Extremely Uncomfortable |

FATIGUE:

| No Fatigue | 1 | 2 | 3 | 4 | 5 | Severe Fatigue |

THERAPIST FEEDBACK

Patient Responses: _____

_____

_____

Massage techniques used: _____

_____

Length of session: _____   Time of rating: ____:____ am pm

Appendix D-2

MASSAGE PATIENT DATA FORM

PART A:

Patient Name _____ Age _____ Sex _____

Unit: _____ Room _____ Nurse _____ Today's Date _____

Dx _____ Dx Procedure _____

Chemo: Y N   Radiation: Y N   Surgery _____ Date of surg. _____

SENSORY IMPAIRMENT: _____ blind _____ HOH _____ speech

POSITION RESTRICTIONS: SITE RESTRICTIONS:

_____ no walking   _____ lay flat   _____ ostomy   _____ rash
_____ elevate extremity _____ logroll   _____ incision   _____ dressing
_____ posture   _____ open wound   _____ infection
                                        changes   _____ IV site   _____ drain
                                                        _____ tumor site   _____ trach
PSYCHOSOCIAL: _____ bone mets   _____ foley

_____ lonely   _____ unalert   PRESSURE RESTRICTIONS: Y N
_____ confused   _____ disoriented
_____ depressed   _____ DVT   _____ heparin
                                                        _____ thrombocytopenia _____ neutropenia

PART B:

Have they ever received a professional massage?   Y N

What would the patient like from the massage session?
Subjective -

Check if the patient has any of the following conditions:
_____ diabetes   _____ varicose veins   _____ easy bruising   _____ scars
_____ contagious disease _____ joint swelling   _____ arthritis   _____ osteoporosis
_____ high blood pressure _____ heart disease   _____ allergies   _____ headaches
other: _____

PART C: SOAP NOTES

Objective:

Action:

Progress:

Length of session: _____

Appendix D-3

Appendix E
Resources

ORGANIZATIONS

CANCER ORGANIZATIONS

American Cancer Society (ACS). 1-800-227-2345, National Headquarters: 1599 Clifton Rd. N.E., Atlanta GA, 30329. (http://www.cancer.org/) The ACS supports research, offers educational programs, and provides patient and family services.

Anti-cancer Council of South Australia. 618-82914111. http://www.acf.org.au/index2.html or http://www.acf.org.au/cafacts.htm

Anti-cancer Council of Victoria (Australia). 613-92791129. http://www.accv.org.au/1home/home.html

BACUP (British). 0800-181199. medweb.bham.ac.uk/cancerhelp

Camp Good Day and Special Times, Inc. 1-800-785-2135. This non-profit organization provides camping experiences in upstate New York for children and women with cancer or survivors of cancer. The ACS can provide the names of many other camps.

Canadian Cancer Society. (416) 961-7223, National Office: 10 Alcorn Ave., Suite 200, Toronto, Ontario M4V 3B1. (http://www.cancer.ca)

Cancer Information Services (CIS). 1-800-422-6237 (4-CANCER). CIS is a telephone service of the National Cancer Institute that provides information to patients and their families, the public, and health care professionals. Free booklets can also be ordered. Request the "Publications for Cancer Patients and the Public."

CANCER LINK (British). 0800-132905. cancerlink@canlink.demon.co.uk

Cancer Treatment Centers of America. 1-800-234-0497. These centers provide a holistic approach to cancer treatment that includes medical treatment, diet planning, herbal and vitamin supplements, counselling, and other alternative modalities, including massage at some centers.

Commonweal. PO Box 316, Bolinas, CA 94924. 415-868-0970. A retreat center on the California coast for people with cancer. The week-long retreats include yoga, massage, art therapy, support groups, and education.

Imperial Cancer Research Fund. 61 Lincoln's Inn Fields, London WC2A 3PX. (http://www.icnet.uk)

National Association of Breast Cancer Organizations. 1180 Avenue of the Americas, 2nd Floor, New York, NY 10036. Provides information on breast cancer.

National Cancer Institute (NCI). Bldg. 31, 9000 Rockville Pike, Bethesda, MD 20892.
CancerNet—http://wwwicic.nci.nih.gov/
CancerLit—http://wwwicic.nci.nih.gov/canlit/canlit.htm

PDQ. This is a computerized database developed by the National Cancer Institute. It is designed for doctors to quickly access the latest information on prevention, diagnosis, treatment, and rehabilitation; clinical trials that are open for enrollment, and the names of doctors and organizations involved in cancer care. The latest treatment information for most types of cancer is also available by fax at 301-402-5874. Patients can access the same information through CIS at 1-800-4CANCER.

Potentiality, Inc. 16869 SW 65th Ave., #303, Lake Oswego, OR 97035. (503)612-1720. A non-profit organization dedicated to educating people with cancer about alternative and complementary healing modalities.

TOUCH ORGANIZATIONS

Care Through Touch Institute. 2401 LeConte Ave., Berkeley, CA 94709. 510-548-0418. Offers weekend workshops, certification programs, and supervised pastoral internships in the use of massage and touch as ministry for the poor, homeless, elderly, dying, handicapped, those in recovery, and survivors of abuse. Massage is approached as "the art of anointing".

Compassionate Touch. 20 Swan Court, Walnut Creek, CA 94596. 510-935-3906. Offers training programs and videos for working with the elderly, the ill, and the dying.

National Association of Nurse Massage Therapists. PO Box 1150, Abita Springs, LA 70420. 1-888-4NAMT6 or 504-892-6990.

Service Through Touch Educational Resources. 41 Carl St., San Francisco, CA 94117. 415-564-1750. Offers audio and video cassettes and workshops for providing touch to the seriously ill.

Touch Research Institute. University of Miami School of Medicine, Dept. of Pediatrics, PO Box 016820 (D-820), Miami, FL 33101; 305-547-6781; 305-243-6488 (Fax). Published studies are available free of charge. At present two cancer related studies are in progress, one in pediatric oncology and the other with breast cancer patients.

OTHER ORGANIZATIONS

Chalice of Repose Project. Therese Schroeder-Sheker. St. Patrick's Hospital, 554 W. Broadway, Missoula, MT 59802. Dedicated to providing prescriptive music to ease the dying experience.

The Institute for the Study of Health and Illness. PO Box 316, Bolinas, CA 94924. 415-868-2642. Provides instruction for health care providers who wish to develop retreats and support groups for people with life-threatening illness. The workshops are held at Commonweal.

National Family Caregivers Association. 800-896-3650.
info@nfcacares.org or http://www.nfcacares.org

National Hospice Organization. 1901 Moore St., Suite 901, Arlington, VA 22209.

Upaya. 1404 Cerro Gordo, Santa Fe, NM 87501. 505-986-8518. (www.rt66.com/~upaya). Upaya's focus is on spiritually assisted dying.

PUBLICATIONS

RECOMMENDED BODYWORK BOOKS

Barne tt, L. and M. Chambers. *Reiki Energy Medicine: Bringing Healing Touch into Home, Hospital, and Hospice*. Rochester, VT: Healing Arts Press, 1996.

Eos, N. *Reiki and Medicine*. Self-published. White Feather Press, 1995. Author can be contacted at P.O. Box 569, Grass Lakes, MI 49420.

Henderson, J.S. *The Healing Power of Attunement Therapy: Stories and Practice*. Tallahassee FL: Findhorn Press, 1998.

Gordon, R. *Your Healing Hands: The Polarity Experience*. Berkeley, CA: Wingbow Press, 1984.

Motz, J. *Hands of Life*. New York: Bantam, 1998.

Nelson, D. *Compassionate Touch: Hands-On Caregiving for the Elderly, the Ill and the Dying*. Barrytown, NY: Station Hill Press, 1994.

Ray, B. *The 'Reiki' Factor in The Radiance Technique*. Radiance Associates. 1992. Contact: Radiance Associates, PO Box 86425, St. Petersburg, FL 33738.

Wager, S. *A Doctor's Guide to Therapeutic Touch*. New York: Perigee Books, 1996.

RELATED BODYWORK PUBLICATIONS

"Comfort Massage for the Seriously Ill". Contact: Information for People. PO Box 1876, Olympia, WA 98507. 800-754-9790. An informational brochure for clients. Also available is a brochure called "Therapeutic Massage for the Elderly and Ill". Free samples are available.

Dunn, T. and M. Williams. *Massage Therapy Guidelines for Hospital and Home Care*. 1996. Available from: Planetree, 130 Division, Derby, CT 06418.   203-732-1365.

Gibson, K. *Developing a Hospital-Based Massage Therapy Program*. 1992. 1024 Pitkin Ave., Glenwood Springs, CO 81601.   970-945-3060.

Hospital-based Massage Network Newsletter. 5 Old Town Square, Suite 205, Fort Collins, CO 80524. 970-407-9232 or 970-225-9217 (Fax).

Journal of Soft Tissue Manipulation (JSTM). Ontario Massage Therapy Association. 365 Bloor St. E, Suite 1897, Toronto, Ontario, Canada M4W 3L4. 416-968-6487 or 1-800-668-2022 (Canada only). JSTM focuses on research, treatment contraindications and precautions, technique papers, and philosophical issues that relate to medically oriented massage.

Roche, C. *The Insurance Reimbursement Manual: For America's Bodyworkers, Body-therapists and Massage Professionals*. 5th ed. Available through: The Bodytherapy Business Institute, 4157 El Camino Way, Suite C, Palo Alto, CA 94306. 1-800-888-1515.

"The Lives We Touch: Moments that go Beyond Words". This video is about touch in the hospital. Available through Benchmark Publishing Co., 319 10th Ave., PO Box 67, New Glarus, WI 53574-0067. 800-475-4545. 608-938-1717 (Fax).

OTHER SUGGESTED READING ON HEALING, ILLNESS, AND DYING

Barasch, M. *The Healing Path: A Soul Approach to Illness.* New York: Arkana, 1993.

Bernard, J. and M. Schneider. *The True Work of Dying: A Practical and Compassionate Guide to Easing the Dying Process.* New York: Avon Books, 1996

Bolen, J. S. *Close to the Bone: Life-Threatening Illness and the Search for Meaning.* New York: Scribner, 1996.

Callahan, M. and P. Kelly. *Final Gifts.* New York: Bantam Books, 1992.

Caposella, C. and S. Warnock. *Share the Care: How to Organize a Group to Care for Someone Who Is Seriously Ill.* New York: Fireside Books, 1995.

Duda, D. *A Guide to Dying at Home.* John Muir Publications. 1982.

Huddleston, P. *Prepare for Surgery, Heal Faster: A Guide of Mind-Body Techniques.* Cambridge, MA: Angel River Press.

Kornfield, J. *A Path with Heart.* New York: Bantam Books, 1993.

Levine, S. *Guided Meditations, Explorations and Healings.* New York: Anchor Books/Doubleday, 1991.

____ *Healing into Life and Death.* New York: Anchor Books/Doubleday, 1987.

____ *Meetings at the Edge: Dialogues with the Grieving and the Dying, the Healing and the Healed.* New York: Anchor Books/Doubleday, 1984.

____ *Who Dies? An Investigation of Conscious Living and Conscious Dying.* Anchor Books/Doubleday. 1982.

Mindell, A. *Coma: Key to Awakening.* Boston: Shambala, 1989.

Nuland, S. *How We Die: Reflections on Life's Final Chapter.* New York: Knopf, 1994.

Remen, R. *Kitchen Table Wisdom: Stories that Heal.* New York: Riverhead Books, 1996.

Siegel, B. *How to Live Between Office Visits.* New York: HarperCollins, 1993.

READING RELATED TO CANCER

Murphy, G.; L. Morris; and D. Lange. *Informed Decisions: The Complete Book of Cancer Diagnosis, Treatment, and Recovery.* New York: Viking/Penguin Books, 1997.

O'Regan, B. and C. Hirshberg. *Spontaneous Remission: An Annotated Bibliography.* Institute of Noetic Sciences. 1993. Order at 1-800-383-1586. Documents thousands of cancer remissions.

Scientific American. *What You Need to Know About Cancer.* 1996; 275(3). Back issues can be ordered through: Scientific American, Dept. CNCR; 415 Madison Ave., New York, NY 10017-1111. The cost is $5.95.

Steingraber, S. *Living Downstream: An Ecologist Looks at Cancer and the Environment.* Reading, MA: Addison Wesley, 1997.

Swirsky, J. and D. Nannery. *Coping with Lymphedema.* Garden City Park, NY: Avery, 1998.

Appendix F
Glossary of Bodywork Modalities

Chapters 4 and 5 contain detailed information regarding cautions and indications for touch. The Glossary of Bodywork Modalities should be used in conjunction with those chapters. If a person has active cancer or is recovering from treatment, obtain physician approval to administer techniques that apply pressure or movement. Manipulation, massage, or pressure should not be performed at the site of a tumor.

Although most bodywork sessions are performed on a padded table or a floor mat, they can usually be adapted for patients who are in a hospital bed. Many modalities are received unclothed. However, most bodyworkers allow the massage recipient to leave their underwear on, or even receive massage in shorts. If the client completely disrobes, she will be draped with a sheet or towel and only the part being massaged will be exposed.

ACUPRESSURE has its roots in the Chinese medical system and is closely related to acupuncture. In this philosophy, the body contains hundreds of small energy centers, or acu-points, close to the surface arranged along energy channels referred to as meridians. Putting pressure on these points can either activate the "chi," which translates to "life-force energy," or drain excess chi. Disease is believed to be the result of a disturbance in the flow of chi, and re-establishing the flow stimulates the body's ability to heal itself. Acupressure practitioners use a gentle but deep finger pressure. Clients receive sessions while fully dressed, on a floor mat or massage table. Because people with cancer often bruise easily, only a very light pressure should be used. Recipients find these sessions to be both stimulating and relaxing, which can ease the fatigue that accompanies cancer and its treatment. Also see "Shiatsu."

AMMA is the traditional massage of Japan and is the forerunner of Shiatsu. It is based on the principles of traditional Chinese medicine. Amma is not just a method for providing relaxation, but also includes diagnosis and treatment for illness. Stroking and pressure on the points along the energy pathways are used in addition to specialized stretching, kneading, and percussion. See "Shiatsu" and "Acupressure."

ASTON-PATTERNING® is best known as a form of movement re-education. However, it also includes fitness training, ergonomics, and bodywork. The strokes used in the bodywork component can be useful for people with cancer. Aston massage can be received purely for the relaxation value. Other strokes, called Myokinetics, can be used after the client is cancer free to stretch and release fascia, which is beneficial for people affected by adhesions or restrictions in the fascia due to surgery or other injuries. Sessions are given on a massage table. Clients often disrobe down to their underwear or wear shorts and a T-shirt. Massage cream may be used.

ATTUNEMENT THERAPY is a Western healing arts practice with a spiritual basis. Through this modality one's outer being is unified to the inner Source by balancing and clarifying the life force at Reflexology and Vibrational Gateway Points through the etheric body. Focusing energy specifically at the cervical vertebrae and endocrine system, Attunement Therapy brings about balance, clarification, and healing at all levels of being. Practitioners offer non-directed prayer during sessions and are often called upon to be present prior to, during and after surgeries. Attunement practice includes self-attunement, long distance methods, radiant gatherings (prayer circles), and may include the use of symbolic objects. Sessions are received clothed and may be adapted for use on a massage table, chair, or bed. All cancer patients can benefit from Attunement Therapy at any stage of health.

AYURVEDIC MASSAGE is one part of a healing system based on ancient Hindu theory. Generally massage is not given on its own, but is a component of a comprehensive treatment regimen that also includes the use of herbalized steams, diet, Yoga, meditation, breathing exercises, and detoxification routines. Ayurvedic practitioners seek to assist the patient in creating a unity consciousness. Fighting disease is not the focus, the aim is to rebalance the physiology. Copious amounts of herbalized oil are used in the massage session. For the person with cancer, specific sets of stroke patterns would be used to strengthen the immune and nervous systems.

BINDEGEWEBMASSAGE, also known as connective tissue massage, was developed in the 1930's in Germany. Despite being known as connective tissue massage, it actually works with the nerves. Elisabeth Dicke's technique applies brisk, non-painful strokes to the fascia that lies between the skin and muscle. This layer of fascia, or connective tissue, contains many nerve endings which are believed to reflex to, or be associated with, certain pathways of the nervous system and organs. These pathways create zones that are referred to as dermatomes. In Europe, Bindegewebmassage is prescribed for many conditions: asthma, orthopedic and structural problems, colitis, Parkinson's disease, circulatory disorders, and uterine infections, to name some. Sessions are generally received unclothed. However, recipients may wear a gown to insure their modesty is protected. Clients are positioned in a sitting position, with the exception of the legs, which are massaged lying down. No lubricant is used. Cancer patients who are experiencing fatigue may benefit from the stimulating, energizing effect. It also may help the person who has been sedentary to re-establish greater nerve functioning, thereby stimulating organs and muscles.

The BOWEN TECHNIQUE is the invention of Australian Tom Bowen. Mirka Knaster compares practitioners of his modality to piano tuners because of the way they gently pluck tendons, nerves, and muscle fascia. Joints are freed, muscles relaxed, the functioning of the blood and lymph systems improved, and the energy and organ systems are balanced. None of the usual massage strokes, such as pounding, stroking, or pressing, are used. Sessions are given without oil on a massage table. The clothes can be kept on. Because of its gentle nature, the Bowen Technique can be used at all stages of the cancer experience.

COMPASSIONATE TOUCH,® developed by Dawn Nelson, is a therapeutic modality for relating to elderly and/or ill individuals. It combines one-on-one focused attention, gentle touch, and other relaxation techniques with communication skills such as active listening, reflective feedback, and positive instruction. All cancer patients would benefit from receiving this modality. Sessions may be received in a hospital bed, chair, or on a massage table. Recipients can remain clothed or partially clothed or may completely disrobe.

CRANIALSACRAL THERAPIES work to balance the flow of the cerebrospinal fluid in order to restore optimum functioning to the central nervous system and ultimately the entire body. The practitioner uses gentle compressions to realign bones and soft tissue in the skull, mouth, face, vertebral column, and sacrum, thereby allowing the cerebrospinal fluid to flow freely. While these therapies can be used to resolve specific maladies such as headaches, neck and back pain, or balance problems, they also are useful in freeing accumulated stress, which is beneficial to patients at any time. Because of its gentleness, this modality can be used at all stages of the cancer experience. Sessions are given on a massage table and can be received clothed or unclothed.

ESALEN MASSAGE was developed by practitioners at the Esalen Institute in Big Sur, California. This technique aims to relax by blending the long, flowing, gliding strokes of Swedish Massage with light rocking, passive joint movement, and deeper tissue work, if appropriate. Esalen Massage conveys a better. Reflexologists apply a deep pressure with the thumbs. Modification in pressure may be needed for people with cancer, depending on what stage they are in. Reflexology is especially useful for conditions in which massage directly to an area is inadvisable or not tolerated by the patient, such as constipation or a surgical site.

REIKI is a Japanese word that roughly translated means "universal life force." It is a method of natural healing designed to strengthen a person's absorption of universal life energy (similar to chi). This technique is non-manipulative and works with or without touch, as necessary. It balances and aligns the body's energy and energy field, systematically teaches people how to access and use universal energy for stress management and personal growth, and helps the body, mind, emotions, and spirit regain balance. Practitioners serve as a conduit to universal life energy and may transmit it directly to clients by giving hands-on treatments or by conducting it through "distance healing." One way to describe the hands-on sessions is as sacred touch. Sessions are given with the recipient being clothed and consist of a series of hand positions that begin at the head and systematically work toward the feet. A pressureless touch with no movement or stroking is used. Recipients find the sessions to be calming, nurturing, and undemanding. Reiki is an excellent modality for people with cancer, especially during the treatment phase, following surgery, or at times when it is inadvisable to apply strokes that increase circulation or use pressure, such as with thrombocytopenia or deep vein thrombosis. In addition to being useful as a hands-on technique, Reiki also can be beneficial for situations in which the practitioner is unable to be with the patient, such as in the operating room, during procedures, or if the practitioner lives in another city. This "distance healing," which some liken to prayer, is useful during these times. Another feature of Reiki is that it can be self-administered and is extremely simple. Anyone can learn to be a practitioner, even children. Many other systems have been formed around the Reiki modality, such as The Radiance Technique and Mariel.

ROLFING,® originally known as Structural Integration, was developed by biochemist Ida Rolf, and has been a springboard for several other structural approaches. Rolfer Kerry Haladae describes it as a "technique for reordering the whole body." Rolf understood that traumas, poor posture, and emotional stress caused the fascia to become misaligned, forcing compensation at secondary sites in the body, and creating a structure that had a poor relationship to gravity. A person's relationship to gravity, Rolf believed, affected behavior and ability to function. Deep manipulation is applied to the muscles and fascia to achieve correct body alignment for that person. Although the ten session series focuses mainly on the body, the body and mind are considered to be one, with Rolfing improving both. Clients are attracted to this system to increase body awareness, to address physical and emotional pain, to enhance athletic performance, or as a path to personal growth. Rolfing has a reputation for being painful. In the past this may have been true, but less invasive techniques are now taught and practiced, making sessions more comfortable to receive. Each session emphasizes a different area of the body. Treatments are received unclothed on a massage table. Because this system of bodywork can be physically deep and can trigger profound emotional release, cancer patients should wait until they are physically and emotionally healed from their disease. The student clinic at the Rolf Institute has a policy of waiting 18 months.

ROSEN METHOD® is a simple, non-invasive approach that utilizes gentle touch and verbal communication to explore physical and emotional contraction. Marion Rosen believed that a person's musculature and breath are guides to the emotional state and that emotional release and muscular release are interdependent. Her methods can result in increased awareness, emotional release, relaxation, increased self-awareness, decreased pain, profound personal growth, and a breathing pattern that moves more freely. Sessions are given on a massage table.

RUBENFELD SYNERGY METHOD® is an approach to integrate body, mind, and emotions. Originator Ilana Rubenfeld believes that physical and emotional symptoms cannot be separated and must be dealt with simultaneously. She combines touch with verbal expression, visualization, sound, movement, breath, and humor to access emotions and memories stored in the body. Generally sessions are conducted on a massage table, but clients may also sit, or move around the room.

RUSSIAN MASSAGE (KURASHOVA METHOD) is a common, well-accepted form of treatment in Russian hospitals, clinics, and wellness resorts. The strokes administered in this technique look similar to those used in Swedish Massage. The focus, however, is not on the anatomical structure as with most bodywork therapies, but is on the body's physiology. According to Zhenya Wine of the Kurashova Institute, Russian Massage is based on the idea that the body is its own best healer, and "that massage can teach the body how to heal itself." Soviet physicians developed this form of treatment to solve post WWII health problems and have performed 80 percent of the world's massage research. The Kurashova Method is used to treat many dysfunctions such as neuralgia, scoliosis, arthritis, fractures, and tendon or ligament damage. In many cases, patients are able to replace drugs with these massage techniques. It is also given for relaxation, to enhance athletic performance, and to energize the body. The strokes, which are painless and non-invasive, can be applied gently or deeply, as needed, and therefore can be adapted to any stage of cancer. Sessions are given on a massage table, generally with the client unclothed.

SEATED CHAIR MASSAGE, also known as on-site massage, generally focuses on the recipient's head, neck, back, and arms. The client sits/kneels on a padded chair specially designed to support the face, chest, and arms. The massage is usually 10-20 minutes in length and is given through the clothing, using such techniques as compression, acupressure, petrissage, and stretching. Chair massage is especially helpful in the hospital for family caregivers. The practitioner should always check to be sure recipients are not prone to easy bruising.

SHEN, an acronym for Specific Human Energy Nexus, aims to clear emotions trapped within the body by applying gentle touch in a pattern that follows the body's energy flows. When painful emotions, traumas, and memories are held in the body, normal functioning is disrupted, causing psychosomatic conditions such as eating disorders, irritable bowel syndrome, or headaches. Releasing these emotions can re-establish a higher level of physical health. SHEN is useful for such stress-related conditions as depression and anxiety, both of which plague people with cancer. Richard Pavek, SHEN's originator, also purports it to decrease pain and "reduce local swelling by releasing tensions in the surrounding tissues so that drainage can occur." (Knaster, 1996) This is an excellent modality for people with cancer because it can be performed at all stages. Clients receive sessions while clothed.

SHIATSU is a cousin of acupressure, Jin Shin Do, and Amma massage. In Japanese it means "finger pressure." However, the hands, elbows, or knees may also be used on the acu-points along the meridians. This technique aims to balance the flow of vital life energy, or ki. (Ki is the Japanese word for chi.) Shiatsu is a synthesis of modern information from Western anatomy and physiology and the principles of traditional Japanese massage. It's purpose is not just relaxation, but as a tool to treat disease. Different styles of Shiatsu are practiced, each with its own emphasis. Some focus on the meridians, others with the neuromuscular system. Buddhist philosophy, breathing practices, and exercises to stimulate ki are features in various schools of Shiatsu. Stretching and range of motion are usually involved. The same benefits can be achieved for people with cancer through Shiatsu as with acupressure or Jin Shin Do, and the same precautions are in effect. Sessions are generally performed on a floor mat with the client clothed.

SOMATOEMOTIONAL RELEASE (SER) is based on the belief that our bodies hold the energy of past physical and emotional traumas. John Upledger, the originator of this system and CranioSacral Therapy (CST), coined the term "energy cysts" for those areas of congestion which disrupt the body's healthy functioning. Release of these energy cysts occurs as part of a CranioSacral Therapy treatment. In a letter to me, Dr. Upledger reported that he has used both CST and SER with cancer patients for 25 years.

SOMA NEUROMUSCULAR INTEGRATION, or Soma Bodywork, sprang from the work of Ida Rolf. The creators, Bill and Ellen Williams, have refined the strokes used in Rolfing to be less invasive. Such techniques as journal keeping, dialogue, and deep relaxation training are also incorporated. See "Rolfing."

SOMATOSYNTHESIS was developed by chiropractor Cyde Ford from a psychological therapy known as Psychosynthesis. Ford's system incorporates a variety of hands-on techniques, dialogue, and awareness and imagery exercises. The purpose is to help the client gain insight into his physical and psychological states. As with other body-centered psychotherapies, somatosynthesis emphasizes "listening to the body". For many people, just talking is not enough to provide understanding about their psychology, accessing the wisdom of the body is necessary as well. With proper modification, hands-on work can be administered for all people with cancer.

SWEDISH MASSAGE is the most commonly practiced bodywork modality in the West. Long, gliding strokes (effleurage) or rhythmical, kneading strokes (petrissage) form the basis of the sessions. Three other strokes are also included in this system, friction, vibration, and tapping. Swedish Massage sessions are designed to produce relaxation and increase circulation, which helps the body flush out toxins and bring fresh nutrients to the tissues. In addition, it can be used for stimulation, rehabilitation, and recovery from strains and trauma. Effleurage is one of the staples of a bodyworker who massages people with cancer. This stroke can be modified to fit almost any situation with the exception of deep vein thrombosis and very low platelet levels. The client generally receives Swedish Massage unclothed on a padded table. The body is draped with a towel or sheet, only the part being massaged will be exposed. Oil or lotion is applied to facilitate the rhythmical, gliding motion.

THAI MASSAGE, the ancient form of massage from Thailand, can best be described as a combination of acupressure and yoga. According to its theory, 72,000 lines of energy run throughout the body and on these lines acupressure points are found. However, only ten of these channels, or Sen, are focused on in Thai Massage. Working on the Sens removes blockages, allowing energy to flow freely. Pressure is applied to them generally with the thumbs and palms, but feet, forearms, elbows, and knees may also be used. Yoga stretches are an integral part of Thai Massage and are performed with the help of the practitioner. In addition to clearing energy pathways, this system can calm the nerves, increase circulation, stimulate organs, energize and relax muscles, and improve range of motion. Sessions are conducted on a floor mat with the client clothed. People in fragile health may be able to tolerate a greatly modified version of the acupressure component, but should not participate in the vigorous stretching or allow deep pressure.

THERAPEUTIC TOUCH (TT) is based on the idea that our energy extends beyond the skin into an "energy field" that surrounds and interpenetrates the body. Illness is believed to be influenced by imbalances or blockages in the energy field, also known as the aura. TT aims to assist the physical body by attuning the energy field around it. Practitioners generally do not touch the body, but work with the hands in the energy field. Re-establishing proper energy flow then allows the individual's own healing powers to take over. Because this modality is not administered directly to the body, it can be given at all stages of illness and may be especially helpful for situations in which touch is not tolerated by the patient or is inadvisable, as in the case of bone metastases, incisions, or deep vein thrombosis.

TOUCH FOR HEALTH uses muscle testing, also known as applied kinesiology, to discover blockages in the muscles and meridians. Acupressure and massage techniques are used to improve postural balance, decrease pain, and create relaxation. See "Acupressure" for cautions.

Appendix F-7

TRAGER PSYCHOSOCIAL INTEGRATION® is the creation of Milton Trager, M.D. Dr. Trager taught that the mind is the source of pain, rigid movement, and dysfunction, and that by releasing the body's holding patterns, the mind also will be liberated. These holding patterns may have developed as a reaction to emotional injury, surgery, an accident, or disease. The trademark of a Trager session is a gentle, steady, rhythmical rocking by the practitioner, which seeks to impart a sense of lightness and freedom to the client's unconscious mind. Deep relaxation, increased mobility, greater energy, and inner peace are created. The body is re-minded of feeling open and free. Trager's work also includes a series of movement exercises called Mentastics which the client performs at home to reinforce the feelings gained during the hands-on session. During his life, Dr. Trager was able to improve the health of people with a variety of neuromuscular disorders, such as multiple sclerosis, Parkinson's disease, polio, and stroke. With proper adaptation, Trager could be used with most cancer patients who are in treatment or recovering from it. The gentle movements would help the patient let go of the fear accumulated in the body over months or years of treatment, improve functioning in areas affected by surgery, and increase energy and vitality. Sessions are conducted on a massage table and can be received clothed or unclothed.

TRIGGER POINT THERAPY is a generic term for the variety of bodywork modalities used to release tender areas in the muscles which can be felt as lumps or knots. These sensitive areas are known as trigger points (TP) because they cause pain to radiate to other parts of the body. Trigger point therapies, such as Neuromuscular Therapy and Bonnie Prudden's Myotherapy, use a deep, sustained pressure with the fingers, knuckles, and elbows. Stretching exercises are used following the release of a TP. Practitioners must be mindful of the amount of pressure applied to people with cancer or recovering from treatment because they often bruise easily. Treatments are given on a massage table and can be used through clothing or on bare skin. A lubricant is not used. Surgical patients, especially post-mastectomy patients, may benefit from an increase in range of motion and a decrease in localized pain as a result of trigger point therapy.

ZERO BALANCING® (ZB), created by Fritz Smith, M.D., is a method of gentle touch used to align the body's skeletal structure with its flow of energy. Western concepts of anatomy, physiology, and kinesiology are brought together with Eastern concepts of energy currents, mechanisms of healing, and anatomy. The goal is not to fix or heal but to create a state within the body that will allow well-being and health to arise naturally. Contact with specific bony points is emphasized. One of the underlying beliefs is that bones contain the most dense and unconscious energy, and that one's deepest essence is carried within them. ZB does not diagnose illness nor claim to be a treatment for certain maladies. However, relief from physical and emotional symptoms may occur. Sessions are received clothed, on a padded table. As well as gentle touch, pressing, lifting, pulling, twisting, stretching, and bending may be incorporated into the sessions. Smith advises people with knee replacements to forego Zero Balancing, and those with hip replacements to proceed with care. With proper modification, ZB could be used at any time for the person with cancer. During periods of fragility, it may be best to avoid the lifting, pulling, twisting, and bending, and apply only gentle touch and movements.

REFERENCES

1. Claire, T. *Bodywork: What Type of Massage to Get – And How to Make the Most of It.* New York: William Morrow, 1995.

2. Discover Lymph Drainage Therapy. *International Alliance of Healthcare Educators.* 1996.

3. Haladae, K. *Rolfing* (Educational brochure).

4. Jerome, T. Zero Balancing: Bodywork of Relationship. *Massage Magazine.* Sept./Oct. 1997. p. 35-43.

5. Juhan, D. The Trager Approach: Psychophysical Integration and Mentastics. *The Trager Journal*. Vol. II, 1987.

6. Knaster, M. *Discovering the Body's Wisdom*. New York: Bantam Books, 1996.

7. Krieger, D. *The Therapeutic Touch*. Englewood, NJ: Prentice-Hall, 1979.

8. Kurashova Institute brochure.

9. Myofascial Release. *Myofascial Release Treatment Centers*.

10. Ray, B. *The 'Reiki' Factor in The Radiance Technique*. St. Petersburg, FL: Radiance Associates, 1992.

11. Henderson, J.S. *The Healing Power of Attunement Therapy: Stories and Practice*. Tallahassee FL: Findhorn Press, 1998.

Appendix G

A Summary of the Potential Benefits of Bodywork for Cancer Patients

1. Moisturizes the skin and prevents problems such as bedsores.

2. Relieves muscle soreness due to prolonged bedrest.

3. Increases circulation. Lymphatic flow is stimulated, which helps in the elimination of waste products; vascular flow is also stimulated, bringing fresh nutrients to the area.

4. Increases range of motion.

5. Increases relaxation.

6. Decreases edema and lymphedema.

7. Sedates or stimulates nervous system, depending on the modality used.

8. Encourages deeper respiration.

9. Improves bowel activity.

10. Increases alertness and mental clarity.

11. Improves sleep.

12. Provides pain relief and reduces the need for pain medication.

13. Decreases symptoms related to chemo and radiation such as fatigue, nausea, diarrhea, and loss of appetite.

14. Stimulates faster wound healing.

15. Provides faster recovery from anesthesia.

16. Shortens hospital stays.

17. Increases elasticity to scarred areas.

18. Breaks up adhesions associated with scarring.

19. Increases the effectiveness of other treatments, such as pain medication, physical therapy, or a medical procedure.

20. Increases patient's awareness of stress signals.

21. Decreases anxiety and depression.

22. Provides distraction.

23. Provides relief from isolation.

24. Offers meaningful social interaction.

25. Provides a doorway to greater intimacy with family and friends.

26. Provides relief of touch deprivation.

27. Provides a forum for patients to express their feelings.

28. Re-establishes a positive body image.

29. Gives patient a sense of participation in the healing process.

30. Re-builds hope.

RESOURCES

1. Barnett, L. and M. Chambers. *Reiki Energy Medicine*. Rochester, VT: Healing Arts Press, 1996.
2. Gibson, K. *Developing a Hospital-Based Massage Therapy Program*. Self-published. 1994.
3. Nelson, D. *Compassionate Touch*. Barrytown, NY: Station Hill Press, 1994.
4. Ray, B. *The 'Reiki' Factor in The Radiance Technique*. St. Petersburg, FL: Radiance Associates, 1992.
5. Wager, S. *A Doctor's Guide to Therapeutic Touch*. New York: Perigee Books, 1996.

Index

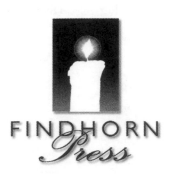

FINDHORN
Press

Findhorn Press is the publishing business of the Findhorn Community which has grown around the Findhorn Foundation in northern Scotland.

For further information about the Findhorn Foundation and the Findhorn Community, please contact:

Findhorn Foundation
The Visitors Centre
The Park, Findhorn IV36 3TY, Scotland, UK
tel 01309 690311• fax 01309 691301
email vcentre@findhorn.org
www.findhorn.org

For a complete Findhorn Press catalogue, please contact:

Findhorn Press

305a The Park,
Forres IV36 3TE
Scotland, UK
Tel 01309 690582
freephone 0800-389-9395
Fax 01309 690036
e-mail info@findhornpress.com
www.findhornpress.com

If you live in the USA or Canada, please send your request to:

Findhorn Press

c/o Lantern Books
One Union Square West, Suite 201
New York, NY 10003-3303
Tel 212-414-2275
Fax 212-414-2412

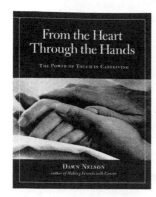

From the Heart Through the Hands:
The Power of Touch in Caregiving
by Dawn Nelson

"This book is a treasure. The author's depth of experience as a healer and meditator shines throughout. Along with books such as *How Can I Help?* by Ram Dass and *Healing into Life and Death* by Stephen Levine, this book leads to greater understanding of life, death, and the true meaning of healing."
—Karen Buhler, M.D.

"Dawn Nelson teaches us the skill of attentiveness in touch and elucidates this gentle interaction that is the connection between our emotions and the other's need. This book demonstrates the art of accurate expression through touch."
—Isaac Cohen, L.Ac, O.M.D., University of California, San Francisco Cancer Center. Author of *Breast Cancer: Beyond Convention*

"In *From the Heart Through the Hands*, Dawn Nelson illustrates how to put the care back into health care! Integrating personal experience and skillful instruction, Dawn teaches the reader how the most basic form of human communication can facilitate physical, emotional and spiritual healing for the caregiver as well as for the patient."
—Irene Smith, Founder, Service Through Touch

"As a medical oncologist, I am well aware of the multiple challenges faced by patients and their support teams in end of life care. I strongly recommend Ms. Nelson's book for hospice team members and all other care providers."
—Dr. John F. Simmons, Jr., Kaiser Permanente Medical Center

This book is for people who feel comfortable communicating through their hands and for those who wish to feel more ease in transmitting care through touch. It is for people whose responsibility or job or gift is to oversee or to help take care of the elderly and ill members of our society. It is for sons and daughters caring for aging parents with physical impairments that effect a role reversal in a lifetime of relating. It is for the courageous men and women who continue caring for spouses or mothers or fathers with dementia related diseases such as Alzheimer's after such a disease has robbed that loved one of the ability to remember the relationship he or she once shared with the caregiver. It is for companions and family members struggling and sometimes sacrificing to provide care for their loved ones at home.

This book is for doctors who have forgotten or never learned that touch is medicine and for those who are wise enough to know that a five-second hug, offered as a gesture of shared humanity, can often do more to assuage fear and anxiety than a five-minute lecture. It is for nurses and nursing assistants who, once trained in giving back rubs to hospitalized patients to reduce discomfort and induce sleep, in current care systems may be more often in contact with equipment than with people, or spend most of their time dispensing medicines and completing paperwork. It is for the restorative aids, the occupational and physical and recreational therapists in extended care facilities who are searching for more effective and affirming ways of relating to those whom they serve. It is for hospice professionals and volunteers, hired companions, geriatric consultants, guardians, home health aids and others who want to help improve quality of life for their charges and clients. It is for chaplains and social workers and grief counselors who wish to reclaim the power of intentional touch in ministering to the frail, the distraught and the bereaved. It is for massage therapy students desiring to build careers in arenas that combine service with professional and personal growth and for practitioners whose hearts and hands lead them to forge new paths in venues where their skills are sorely needed. It is for anyone who wishes to use touch more consciously and compassionately in relating to the elderly, the ill and the dying.

Dawn Nelson is a nationally recognized speaker, author and educator, and the founder of Compassionate Touch® for those in Later Life Stages. The mother of three, Dawn resides with her husband, youngest daughter, and assorted animal companions in Walnut Creek, California. She continues to be interested in improving quality of life for the elderly and the ill, giving Compassionate Touch® training workshops and speaking at Conferences worldwide.

PUBLISHED BY FINDHORN PRESS — SAME FORMAT AND SIZE AS MEDICINE HANDS — ISBN 1-899171-93-2